Ayurvedic Cure

The efficacy and philosophy of Ayurveda, is now accepted by the modern medical community. It takes a holistic view of health, emphasising a balanced diet, physical fitness, healthy lifestyle, hygiene and body care for a disease-free, long and healthy life.

Unlike modern medicine, Ayurveda treats the individual and not merely the disease. In lucid, easy-to-understand language, the book discusses Ayurvedic treatment for almost one hundred diseases: from the common to the more serious; from fevers, constipation, headaches and common cold to insomnia, ulcers, diabetes, impotence and gout. All remedies are based on the inherent healing properties of natural substances—plants, vegetables, fruits, herbs, minerals and trace elements; and are, therefore, safe, effective and affordable.

Dr N. Anjneya Murthy, M.D. (Ayur.), is an Assistant Professor of *Kaya Chikitsa* (General Medicine), teaching post-graduate classes at the Government College of Indian Medicine, Mysore. Before taking up teaching, he was a senior consulting physician in the Department of Ayurvedic Medicine at the prestigious Moolchand Hospital in New Delhi. D.P. Pandey was a researcher and co-author of several popular self-help books on health-related subjects for the layman.

Health Care in
Orient Paperbacks

Magnetic Cure for Common Diseases (*Illus.*)
Yogic Cure for Common Diseases (*Illus.*)
Accupressure Cure for Common Diseases (*Illus.*)
Nature Cure for Common Diseases
Home Guide to Medical Emergencies (*Illus.*)
The Complete Book of Family Homeopathic Medicine (*Illus.*)
The Complete Book of Home Remedies (*Illus.*)
The Complete Family Medicine Book
Mental Tension and Its Cure
A-Z of Childhood Illnesses (*Illus.*)
Aromatherapy (*Illus.*)
Herbal Remedies & Home Comforts
A Guide to Herbal Remedies
Healing with Gems & Crystals

Ayurvedic Cure
for Common Diseases

Dr. N.A. Murthy
D.P. Pandey

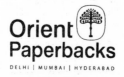

Orient
Paperbacks

DELHI | MUMBAI | HYDERABAD

Disclaimer: This book is designed to provide information in regard to the subject matter covered. The authors and the publisher shall have neither liability nor responsibility to any person or entity with respect to any loss, damage, or injury caused or alleged to be caused directly or indirectly by the information contained in this book. The information presented herein is in no way intended as a substitute for medical counseling.

www.orientpaperbacks.com

ISBN 13: 978-81-222-0180-2
ISBN 10: 81-222-0180-6

1st Published 1982
5th Revised & Enlarged Edition 1995
9th Printing 2005

Ayurvedic Cure for Common Diseases

Cover design by Vision Studio

Published by
Orient Paperbacks
(A division of Vision Books Pvt. Ltd.)
5A/8 Ansari Road, New Delhi-110 002

Printed in India at
Jay Kay Offset Printers, Delhi-110 041

Cover Printed at
Ravindra Printing Press, Delhi-110 006

Preface

Ayurveda–the science of life–has its roots in antiquity and has been practised in our country for centuries. The incursions of Western culture and education put it in eclipse, albeit temporarily, and modern medicine was given the pride of place when invaders from the West followed each other into our land. English and its teaching introduced British ways of thinking, and those educated according to Western standards tended to forget their own heritage. Practitioners of Ayurveda were called quacks, and loss of governmental and even social recognition, at least among the elite, put this ancient science in the shade. It was only after India became free that it was revived.

Modern medicine's preoccupation with germs as causative of diseases and its expertise in killing off those germs has given rise to a serious problem. Each new medicine has created new problems, in that along with the germs responsible for causing morbidity, it also kills the beneficial bacteria that help the human body to maintain its balance. A glance at medical literature published by pharmaceutical companies will show that most medicines have harmful side-effects. Antibiotic drugs are generally administered by allopaths along with certain vitamins because they tend to kill off the bacteria which produce those vitamins in the body. Even so, most practitioners of modern medicine use antibiotics rather indiscriminately, thus creating complications for their patients. Homoeopaths, naturopaths and, of course, Ayurvedic physicians come across myriads of cases which have been complicated due to indiscriminate use of allopathic drugs, finally compelling the patients to turn to alternative systems of medicine.

The present work is intended to inform the general reader about Ayurveda and its efficacy in treating diseases. The method of treatment of the subject is two-fold: though the causative factors of diseases are treated according to Ayurvedic doctrine, modern medical terms have also been used to facilitate the understanding of those who are familiar only with modern medicine. In so far as the drugs used for the treatment of various diseases are concerned, home remedies are also mentioned along with standard Ayurvedic preparations manufactured by Ayurvedic drug houses. Procedures for the manufacture of drugs have not been mentioned since they are a better subject for professional treatises. This is a book for laymen, written by a practising Ayurvedic physician in conjunction with a layman.

Most of the common diseases are dealt with in considerable detail. The authors are sure that if a reader follows the regimen indicated along with the medicines which are readily available, he will stand to benefit. Care must, however, be taken to be sure about the malady from which one suffers. Even though Ayurvedic remedies do not, as a rule, have any harmful side-effects, they have their own properties, and if a malady is caused by the aggravation of *pitta,* the remedy has to be *pittahara;* any other drug would complicate the case, if not exacerbate it.

This is the fifth edition of the book, which has been extensively revised and expanded to explain the theory of Ayurveda and its approach to curing diseases. More diseases have also been included.

The authors have no doubt that readers will find this edition comprehensive and useful.

The Authors

Contents

Publisher's Note

Ayurveda is a complete system of medicine which deals with practically the entire range of diseases and ailments: common and rare, existent and those which have largely been eradicated now. This book, however, deals more with common diseases.

All Sanskrit and Hindi words are italicised. Ayurvedic terms are explained in the Glossary. Suggested medicines and prescriptions are readily available at chemists, Ayurvedic dispensaries and grocery stores.

Index of Diseases

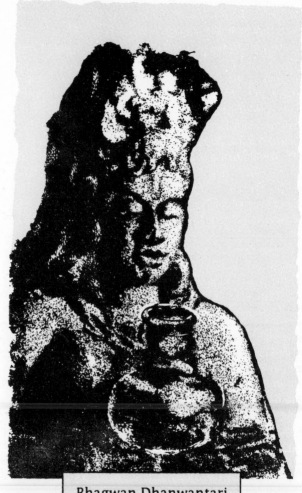

Bhagwan Dhanwantari
God of Ayurveda

Ayurveda—An Overview

हिताहितं सुखं दुःखमायुस्तस्य हिताहितम् ।
मानं च तच्च यत्रोक्तमायुर्वेद: स उच्यते ॥

*That is named Ayurveda (the science of life), wherein are laid
down the good and the bad of life, the happy and unhappy life,
and what is wholesome and what is unwholesome in relation
to life, as also the span of life.*

CHARAKA SAMHITA

AYURVEDA IS a science based on ancient Indian philosophy. It
can appropriately be called 'The Science of Living'. Ayurveda
traces its etymology to *Ayush*, meaning 'life', and *Veda*, which
originates from *vid* or knowledge. Popularly speaking, Ayurveda
can be defined as a medical science which helps the human
body to keep fit, while providing cures from indigenous plants,
animal products and minerals for ailments.

Ayurveda is, essentially, the science of healthy living; it is
as much concerned with the normal as with the abnormal or
pathological. Being essentially a science of healing, it
concentrates on what is required to lead a healthy, normal life.
It deals not only with what is to be done when one falls ill,
but also with what should be done to maintain one's health and
vigour. Ayurveda contains details about body care and the
various foods and drinks which promote health.

Origin of Ayurveda

Even though references to the principles of medicine are
found in most of the *Vedas*, the main body of Ayurveda is found

in the fourth *Veda*—the *Atharva Veda*. However, even though Ayurveda is part of the *Atharva Veda*, it is also recognized as an *upa* or supplementary *Veda* in its own right. It contains the description of various diseases and their aetiology, and recommends the correct diet and behaviour regimen to counter these diseases. Mythology has it that Brahma, the creator, imparted the knowledge of Ayurveda to Prajapati Daksha who, in turn, passed it on to the Ashwinikumara twins who were the physicians to the gods. The Ashwinikumaras then proffered this knowledge to Lord Indra. Dhanwantari was instructed by Lord Indra to spread this invaluable science of longevity on the earth. Sushruta, a renowned surgeon and student of Dhanwantari, wrote his famous compendium on surgery—the *Sushruta Samhita.* To Charaka, who probably lived sometime between the second century B.C. and the second century A.D., goes the credit for the famous treatise on general medicine, the *Charaka Samhita. Charaka Samhita* and *Sushruta Samhita* are the two ancient treatises on which Ayurveda is based.

Basic Principles of Ayurveda

According to ancient Indian philosophy, the universe is composed of five basic elements or *pancha bhutas: prithvi* (earth), *ap*(water), *teja* (fire), *vayu* (air), and *akash* (ether). Everything in the universe, including food and the bodies we possess, is derived from these *bhutas.* A fundamental harmony therefore exists between the macrocosm (the universe) and the microcosm (the individual). As already stated, the human being is comparable to the cosmos, being a miniscule image of the great entity.

The *Pancha Bhuta* Theory and the Human Body: The human body is in a state of continuous flux or dynamic equilibrium. The *pancha bhutas* are represented in the human body as the *doshas, dhatus,* and *malas.*

There are three *doshas* in the body.[1] They are *vata, pitta,* and *kapha.* There are no direct equivalents for these three *doshas,* known as *tridoshas,* in English. However the factors

---

1. The equivalent of the three *doshas* in ancient Greek medicine are the four humours, namely, blood, phlegm, yellow bile, and black bile.

responsible for movement and sensation in a single cell/whole body are the representatives of *vata*. The factors responsible for digestion, metabolism, and energy are the representatives of *pitta*. The factors responsible for strengthening the stomach and the joints, providing firmness to the limbs, and refreshing the sense organs are the representatives of *kapha*. There are some special areas in the body in which each *dosha* predominates, namely, the chest for *kapha*, digestive organs for *pitta*, and the large intestine for *vata*.

The *dhatus* are the body constituents and form the basic structure of the body, each one having its own function. The *dhatus* are seven in number: *rasa* (food juices), *rakta* (haemoglobin portion of the blood), *mamsa* (muscle tissue), *medas* (fat tissue), *asthi* (bone tissue), *majja* (bone marrow), and *shukra* (semen).

Malas are by-products of the *dhatus*, partly used by the body, and partly excreted as waste matter after the process of digestion is over. These play a supporting role while they are in the body, and when they are eliminated, their supporting role is finished. The useful elements absorbed by the body are retained as *prasad* (useful matter), while those excreted are known as *malas* (waste matter). The chief *malas* are *mutra* (urine), *shakrit* (faeces), and *sweda* (perspiration).

The *doshas, dhatus,* and *malas* should be in a state of perfect equilibrium for the body to remain healthy. Any imbalance among these constituents results in ill health and disease.

The *Pancha Bhuta* Theory and the Food We Eat: The food we eat is also composed of the five *bhutas*. Different combinations of the *bhutas* confer different attributes on food. One important attribute is *rasa* (taste)—sweet, sour, saline, pungent, bitter, and astringent. The other attributes are *guna* (virtue), *virya* (potency), and *vipaka* (the taste that arises after the digestion and metabolism of a substance).

As the digestive process begins, the food is acted upon by the *agnis* (various digestive juices) and enzymes.

Branches of Ayurveda

Ayurveda maintains that there is a definite relationship between illness and the metaphysical state of an individual. Its approach to medical treatment is to focus on the person rather than the disease.

Ayurveda has eight distinct branches: *Kayachikitsa*—general medicine; *Shalya tantra*—major surgery; *Shalakya tantra*—ear, nose, throat, eye, and mouth diseases; *Bhuta vidya*—psychiatry; *Bala tantra*—obstetrics, gynaecology, and paediatrics; *Agada tantra*—toxicology; *Rasayana tantra*—rejuvenation; and *Vajikarana tantra*—aphrodisiacs. It is because of this eightfold development that this system of medicine is sometimes called the *Ashtanga Ayurveda*. The present book, however, concerns itself essentially with *Kayachikitsa*, the practice of general medicine.

There are systems which developed out of Ayurveda or were influenced by it. One such system is the Tibetan system of medicine which is the mainstay of the majority of Tibetan people not only in India, but in neighbouring countries too.

Researches in traditional medicine—an epithet which Ayurveda richly deserves—have confirmed the efficacy of most of the natural substances used by the practitioners of Ayurveda: bitter gourd to revive a failing pancreas; papaya seeds to kill intestinal worms without causing harm—these are just two cases in point. The *Charaka Samhita* elaborates on the qualities of these two substances and many more for the amelioration of morbid states.

The Body Constituents & Disease

वातपित्तश्लेष्मणां पुनः सर्वशरीरचराणां सर्वाणि स्रोतांस्ययनभूतानि ।

The Tridoshas—vata, pitta, and kapha—traverse through all the systems of circulation.

CHARAKA SAMHITA

SINCE THE human body and nature are in a state of continuous flux, Ayurveda maintains that a dynamic equilibrium of all the body constituents is imperative for perfect health.

The Theory of the *Tridoshas*

The *Tridoshas,* as introduced in the previous chapter, comprise *vata, pitta,* and *kapha.* They hold the pride of place among the body constituents. It would be relevant here to point out that the *doshas* are not defects as some translators of Ayurvedic texts have erroneously assumed. *Vata* is a combination of two elements of the universe , namely, air and ether. *Pitta* is an amalgam of fire and earth, and *kapha* is the combination of earth and water.

When any of the three *doshas* becomes excessively agitated or increases disproportionately in relation to the others, an imbalance is created, and disease results. The loss of dynamic equilibrium may be due to the excessive or deficient use of, or the misuse of the five sense organs—the ears, skin, eyes, tongue, and nose; action of body, mind, or speech; and time, that is, the different seasons.

19

The restoration of health would then depend on regaining the balance among the three *doshas*. That balance would, in turn, depend on the consumption of environmental matter in the right form, proportion, combination, and at the right time. When the physician becomes sure of the nature of the imbalance of the *doshas,* he prescribes a substance, namely, a drug or a diet which will correct the disequilibrium.

Everything in nature has a relevance for medicine and that is why Ayurveda has collected a fund of data on the therapeutic effect of all kinds of natural substances. Seasons, plants, natural substances, and constituents of the body are all integrated into a complex theory of physical health as an equilibrium of somatic and environmental elements.

Body Constitutions *(Deha-Prakritis)*

The theory of *tridoshas* has led the ancient teachers to make a classification of human constitutions or *deha-prakritis*. The predominance of one *dosha* determines the constitution that a person has. If there is an excess of *vata*—in other words—if the wind is over-agitated, it results in a person having a *vatala* constitution. Likewise, the predominance of the other two *doshas* gives rise to *pittala* or *shleshmala dehaprakriti*. The other four constitutions depend on the vitiation of more than one *dosha*. The *deha-prakritis* are pre-determined body constitutions that a person is born with and there is no change in their basic structure till one dies.

Each type of body constitution or *deha-prakriti* has some peculiar dietary and other habits, and a predictable response to drugs. It is one of the cardinal rules of Ayurveda that medicine cannot be prescribed for a patient unless the physician has taken into account the type of constitution the patient has, because a drug which helps one type of constitution will not help a different *deha-prakriti*. It is imperative to understand that in Ayurveda, the true drug is the one which cures a patient without producing any side-effects. Ayurveda maintains that illness results from the disturbance of the equilibrium among the three *doshas* and other body constituents, and any loss of that balance in an individual makes him/her susceptible to manifold disorders.

The Body Constituents and Their Functions

We have already noted that according to Ayurveda, a lack of balance among the *doshas, dhatus,* and *malas* results in disease. Let us now take a closer look at each of the body constituents.

The *Tridoshas: The Role of Vata.* The normal function of **vata** or *vayu* is to sustain the body, and that is why it is the originator of every kind of action in the body. It has been called the *Tantra-Yantra Dhara*: the one which maintains or keeps the human machinery and its parts in good shape. *Vayu* occupies the pride of place among the three *doshas.* Just as the wind controls the direction of the clouds, so does *vayu* control the functioning of *pitta* and *kapha.*

There are five kinds of *vata* or *vayu: prana, udana, vyana, samana,* and *apana. Prana vayu* is responsible for breathing and the swallowing of food. It is also responsible for the functioning of the heart and the parts of the body directly connected with the heart. Not only does it maintain the functioning of the heart—it also sustains the mind, the senses, the intellect, the arteries, the veins, and the nerves. *Udana vayu* is responsible both for the production of the various sounds and speech, and the action and the effort to keep up the strength of the body, mind, memory, and intellect. *Samana vayu* helps in the action of the digestive enzymes. It separates the essences vital for the nourishment of the body and sends the wastes to the large intestines. *Apana vayu* is situated in the lower part of the digestive tract, the urinary system, and the reproductive organs. Its function is to hold the faeces, urine, menses, and semen upto a normal period, and then to expel them through the various orifices of the body. This *vayu* is one of the most important factors in the body since its proper functioning keeps a person healthy. In an abnormal state, it moves upwards and depresses the diaphragm, giving rise to a sense of acute discomfort. *Vyana vayu* flows through the whole body, carrying the nutrients with it. It helps the excretion of perspiration, and controls the opening and closing of the eye lids, as also other movements of the body.

21

The Role of Pitta. Like the *vayus*, **pittas** are also of five kinds: *pachak, ranjaka, sadhaka, alochaka,* and *bhrajaka. Pachaka pitta* is mainly responsible for the digestion of food. It divides the food juice into the useful and waste parts, and then helps the other four types of *pittas* to function normally in the body. *Ranjaka pitta*, as the very name indicates, adds colour to the food juices when they travel from the stomach to the liver. *Sadhaka pitta* has its seat in the heart and is the finest of all the *pittas*. It helps in the normal functioning of the intellect and memory. *Alochaka pitta* is responsible for the maintenance of normal vision in the eyes. *Bhrajaka pitta* is situated in the skin of the body and is responsible for the normal pigmentation of the skin.

The Role of Kapha. Like the *vayus* and the *pittas*, the **kaphas** are also of five types. The first of these is *kledaka*, which, as its name indicates, is responsible for moistening the food in the stomach. It nourishes the other *kaphas* by its special humid properties. The second *kapha*, the *avalambaka*, has its seat in the thorax, and protects the heart from excessive heat by its cooling influence and gives a special power to the heart. The *bodhaka kapha* moistens any substance which comes in contact with the tongue and helps the individual to recognize the taste of substances ingested. Its seat extends from the root of the tongue to the throat. It plays a part in increasing appetite. The fourth *kapha*, the *tarpaka*, cools the sense organs of sight and hearing. The *shleshaka kapha* is situated in the joints of the body. It maintains them in good order so that the various parts of the body not only remain firm, but also have the flexibility to move.

The *Dhatus*: The *dhatus* are constituents which comprise the basic structure of the body. They are seven in number. They are: *rasa*—essence of food; *rakta*—blood; *mamsa*—muscle tissue; *meda*—fat tissue; *asthi*—bones; *majja*—bone marrow; and *shukra*—sperm in males and ova in females.

Malas or the Wastes of the Body: In addition to the *doshas* and the *dhatus* described above, *malas* (the waste products) are the other constituents of the body. The *malas* are the by-products of the various *dhatus* present in the body. The chief

22

malas are *mutra*—urine; *shakrit*—faeces; and *sweda*—perspiration. Other *malas* are: *pitta*; *purisha sneha* or faecal fat; *prajanan malas* or secretion of the genitalia; and *kha malas* or secretions of the various orifices of the body such as the ear, nose, mouth, and so on. *Malas* play a supporting note while they are in the body. They are eliminated once their supporting role is finished.

The concept of *malas,* both as supportive and excretive products of the body, is important to understand. An example from modern medicine would explain it thus: when red blood cells get old, they are destroyed and may be considered as *malas.* The *malas* perform a supportive function when the iron content of the destroyed red blood cells is reabsorbed and utilised by the body directly, and the biliruben content is passed on as bile by the liver into the duodenum, where it aids the absorption of fats. Thereafter, it is excreted in the faeces as a *mala* or waste product. It is in this way that *malas* perform a dual role.

Factors Responsible for Digestion

The six factors which help digestion, which is the mainstay of health, are: *pachaka pitta* or *agni*; *samana vayu; sneha (unctuous substances like ghee)*; *kledaka (kapha)*; time; and a proper combination of the first five. Our food has the property of taste or *rasa* which is of six types: sweet, sour, salty, pungent, bitter, astringent. The food is subjected to the action of the *bodhaka* and the *kledaka kaphas* in the mouth and the upper part of the stomach. The sweet digestive action (*madhura vipaka*) is followed by the action of the *pitta* (*amla vipaka*); later, the *agni* dries up the waste product which goes into the large intestine (*katu vipaka*).

The Role of Agnis: In addition to the *doshas* and *dhatus,* there are elements known as *agnis.* The principal action of *agni* is to help digestion, absorption, and assimilation with the aid of *vayu.* There are thirteen types of *agnis*: seven *dhatu agnis,* pertaining to the seven *dhatus* of the body; five *bhutagnis,* pertaining to the five *bhutas* or elements; and one *jatharagni,* the digestive fire in the stomach. The last named—*jatharagni*—contained in the *pachaka pitta,* is the root of the *agnis* in the body. Its derangement or loss leads to disease.

23

Diagnosis in Ayurveda

तस्माव्याधीन् भिषग्नुपहतसत्त्वबुद्धिर्हेत्वादिभिर्यथावदनबुद्ध्येत ।

*Therefore the physician who is of sound mind and understanding
should know accurately the diseases from the view-points of
aetiology, symptomatology, etc.*

CHARAKA-NIDANA

THE PRACTITIONERS of Ayurveda may not use the
sphygmomanometer to measure the blood pressure and the
stethoscope to listen to the heart sounds, yet their methods of
examination of the patient and their diagnosis of the disease
are scientific. In fact, diagnosis in Ayurveda is more detailed
and, therefore, more accurate. The texts lay down the various
techniques for diagnosing the various disorders.

Three Stages of Investigation

Investigation is carried out in three stages: case history of
the patient; objective examination; and inference.

Case History of the Patient: The patient is questioned in
detail about his illness and any illnesses his family has suffered
from. A general evaluation is then made in terms of patient's
body constitution, somatic make-up, gastric capacity, and
capacity for exercise according to age.

Objective Examination: The next stage of examination
entails a thorough examination of the patient's nails, eyes, eye

lashes, eye brows, nose, teeth, lips, hands, feet, hair, pupils, urine, faeces, shadow, and skin lustre. The entire body of the patient is then palpatated to find out its normal and abnormal condition. The physician tries to find out whether a particular organ or the entire system is cold or hot, moist or dry, light or heavy, sensitive or insensitive, rough or smooth, rigid or loose, depressed or elevated. Body odours are paid special attention to. Examination of the ears includes listening to the various sounds emanating from the affected organs. This pathological investigation helps in the assessment of the progress of the disease, its aetiological factors, and the probability of curing the disease.

Inference: The third stage is that of inference in which the physician draws his conclusions based on the case history of the patient and the examination he has completed. At this stage, he is in a position to estimate the life expectancy of the patient.

Identifying the Imbalance of the Body Constituents

On completion of his investigation, the physician can also conclude which particular *dosha* is responsible for the state of morbidity in which the patient has been found. Ayurvedic texts provide detailed descriptions of the symptoms which arise from the decrease or increase of the three *doshas*. As Charaka has laid down in his *Samhita:*

> The *tridoshas*, when increased, manifest their characteristic symptoms in proportion to the intensity of their morbidity. When decreased, they cease to manifest their characteristic qualities and when normal, they perform the normal functions of the body.

After determining the imbalance in the equilibrium of the three *doshas*, the Ayurvedist probes deeper still to identify the type of imbalance and describes it in the context of three phases: waning, aggravating, and expanding. The particular season, the country, and other outside factors are also considered.

Practitioners of Ayurveda are keen observers. They also study the state of the body fluids, blood, flesh, fat, bones, marrow, semen, and the vital essence or *oja* which, incidentally, is known as the vital force in the naturopathic system of medicine. They also try to find out whether the disease is curable or not. As Charaka has pointed out:

> The physician who knows the differential diagnosis between the curable and the incurable disease, conditions and begins treatment with full knowledge of the case, in time, obtains success for his effort without fail.

Sushruta has also given his definition of disease:

> The person who has a normal equilibrium of the *tridoshas,* the seven body constituents, and the body's waste products, as well as a normal appetite, and one who is more joyous in body, mind, and spirit is really healthy; and the person, otherwise, is called unhealthy.

Examination of the Pulse

In addition to the investigative procedures mentioned above, an examination of the pulse of the patient is made. The art of reading the pulse has been developed to such an extent in Ayurveda that many practitioners are said to be able to diagnose a disease correctly merely by feeling the pulse of the patient. The rapidity of the rhythm and the volume of the pulse indicates the particular *dosha* from which the patient is suffering. *Bhava Prakash*[1] and *Sarangadhara Samhita*[2] contain details of pulse examination. Pressure is applied to the radial artery below the thumb with three fingers to see whether it is the *vata*, *pitta,* or *kapha* which is responsible for the state of morbidity. A detailed description has been given of the pulse under various conditions of morbidity in these texts.

Examining the State of Digestion

In addition to the above factors, Ayurveda pays attention to the state of the digestion. The condition of the gastric juices tells the physician what state the patient is in. Attention is also paid to the condition in which the various *srotas* or channels

---

1. *Bhava Prakash*—An Ayurvedic text written by Bhava Mishra in the sixteenth century A.D.
2. *Sarangadhara Samhita*—An Ayurvedic text written by Sarangadhara in the twelfth century A.D.

are, because *srotarodha* or blockade of the channels gives rise to disease. For example, the blockade of the bile ducts results in jaundice, while the scanty passage of urine gives rise to an abnormal proportion of urea in the blood.

Psychosomatic Factors Underlying Physical and Mental Disorders

It is only when a detailed diagnosis has been made that the Ayurvedic practitioner ventures to start his treatment. With an accurate diagnosis, the remedy inevitably will also be effective.

Consistent with its belief that there is an interdependence between the mind and the body, Ayurveda professes that any disturbance—physical or mental—must manifest itself, both in the somatic and in the psychic spheres, through the vitiation of the *doshas*. The *acharyas* have postulated that lust, grief, and fear increase the bile content. The vitiation of *vata* destroys the power of the mind and gives rise to fear, grief, and infatuation. The vitiation of phlegm induces lethargy, infatuation, greed, and indiscrimination. Ayurveda recognizes three classes of disease which are, primarily, of mental origin: *unmada*—mental disorders; *apasmara* and *yoshapasmara*—epilepsy and hysteria; *shokaja* and *bhayaja atisar*—diarrhoea caused by grief and fear; *nidranasha*—insomnia; *shokaja* and *kamaja jwara*—fever born out of grief and sexual desire; and mental symptoms, like delusion and insanity induced by alcohol and drugs.

Therapy for the Mind

Ayurvedic treatment for diseases of mental origin is, overwhelmingly, a physiological therapy for the mind because, according to the thesis of psychosomatic identity, *manas* (mind) is influenced by the imbalance of the *doshas* that also disturbs the gross body. The causative factor in mental disorders is believed to be the disturbance and increase in the mental qualities of *rajas* and *tamas*—that is. the good and bad qualities. This increase is ascribed to *ichha* or desire and *dvesha* or animosity, which, when they cross the limits set by the social milieu or mores, excite the *doshas* which lose their mutual balance. Another reason for the disturbance in the *rajas* and *tamas* is the *samskara* (behaviour) of the subtle body, which is inherited from a previous existence, and is a result of unfulfilled longings and unresolved traumas. The treatment of mental disorders in Ayurveda follows the same line as the treatment of bodily disorders. The famous dictum of Charaka applies here too. The great master said:'Purify, pacify, and remove the cause.'

This is, in fact, the watchword of the Ayurvedic system of therapeutics which has been followed in our country for many centuries.

Importance of Body Care & Diet in Ayurveda

षट्त्रिंशतं सहस्राणि रात्रीणां हितभोजन: ।
जीवत्यनातुरो जन्तुर्जितात्मा संमत: सताम् ॥

The disciplined man who takes a wholesome diet lives for a period of 36,000 nights or a hundred years, blessed by good men and free from disease.

CHARAKA SAMHITA

THE ABOVE *shloka* (stanza) from *Charaka Samhita* exemplifies the concern of the masters with the preventive side of medicine. The ancient treatises of Ayurveda contain detailed instructions about personal hygiene and food that promotes health and longevity.

Body Care

Ayurvedic texts contain detailed instructions about body care and personal hygiene. Chewing of various spices and nuts is recommended for clarity of the voice, a pleasing taste, and fresh smell in the mouth. Gargling with sesame oil is said to enhance the strength of the jaws. Sesame oil also gives depth to the voice and even results in the face becoming plump. Regular oiling of the hair and the ears, and periodic oil massages are a part of the normal recommended body care. Massage makes the physique smooth, strong, and charming, and prevents the onslaught of age. Scents and garlands of flowers are said to stimulate the libido, spread fragrance in the body, and enhance longevity and charm.

29

An Indian psychiatrist was surprised to find the following description of a tongue scraper, the like of which he had not seen in use in any other country, in the *Charaka Samhita:*

> Tongue scrapers, which should be curved and not sharp-edged, are to be made of metals like gold, silver, copper, tin, and brass. The dirt deposited at the root of the tongue obstructs expiration and gives rise to a foul smell: so the tongue should be scraped regularly.

Dietetics

Dietetics, or *Pathyapathya,* forms an integral part of Ayurveda. In addition to a general description of foods that promote health and others which should be avoided or taken sparingly, the ancient texts give instructions about foods that should be allowed to the patients according to the nature or severity of the malady, and those which should be banned. Some medicines are to be taken with certain specific foods such as buttermilk or *kanji* (fermented substances). Certain drugs and formulations are administered to the patient in conjunction with certain foods, failing which, the drugs do not have any curative effect.

In the ancient texts, no section on any disease is complete unless the *pathyapatha* is discussed. The *acharyas* (teachers) knew the specific qualities of the foods and their curative value, and when they were given in conjunction with the drugs, they helped to cure the patient quicker than it would have been possible if those foods had not been given.

In the compendia of Charaka, Sushruta, Vagabhata and others, separate chapters are devoted to the various foods and their effect on the human body. Both vegetarian and non-vegetarian foods have been discussed and recommended for the various physical states. Non-vegetarian diets are particularly recommended in diseases like consumption where the wasting of the flesh is evident and the body has to be repaired by strengthening the *mamsa dhatu.*

The *Rasa* Theory: Explanations and theories about the digestion and assimilation of food in the body are contained in the ancient Indian medical texts. These appear to be far more coherent and advanced when compared with the theories put forward by other modern systems of medicine. One such theory is that of *Rasa* (taste) which occupies a central place in Ayurveda.

According to this theory, the food that we take is composed ultimately of the five elements (*Pancha bhutas*). Different combinations of these *Pancha bhutas* confer different qualities upon different foods. One of the most important of such qualities is that of *rasa*, which may be any one of the following six; sweet, sour, saline, pungent, bitter, and astringent; or a combination of these. Thus, the predominance of water results in a sweet taste; the predominance of earth and fire account for an acid taste; a higher concentration of water and fire lead to a saline taste; a predominance of air and fire provide a hot and pungent taste; an excess of air and *akasa* lend a bitter taste; while air and earth render an astringent taste to food.

Each of these *rasas* is capable of producing certain physiological effects. A sweet taste is said to increase blood, flesh, fat, marrow, semen, and life, while sharpening the six senses. An acid taste is said to facilitate digestion, develop the body and remove *vata*. A saline taste is digestive; it removes *vata*, and secretes *kapha*. A pungent taste provokes digestive fire. A bitter taste promotes the appetite, assists digestion of undigested food, and removes harmful *doshas*. An astringent taste restores balance among the *doshas*.

The Importance of Diet: The emphasis that Ayurveda lays on the diet of the patient is apparent from an old dictum: 'The patient does not require any medicine if he has a wholesome diet and he does not require any medicine either, if he is not on a wholesome diet.' If a person's diet is wholesome, he will not need any medicine because he will not fall ill, and if the diet is faulty, he will not require any medicine because it will not help him without a proper diet. In this connection, one is reminded of the story of the Ayurvedic physician who advised a patient suffering from stomach ache to have his eyes treated. Though the patient was surprised at being advised to have an eye check-up for a stomach ache, the advice was correct because the patient had admitted that the stomach ache had started after he had eaten a burnt *chapatti*. Had he not committed that indiscretion, he would not have suffered from the malady!

The Role of *Pancha Karma*

का कल्पना पंच्सु कर्मसुक्ता ।
क्रमश्चच क:, किं च कृता कृतेषु ॥

What is the method laid down in the five purificatory procedures?
What is the order in which they are to be performed?

THE TERM *Pancha karma* comprises two words: *pancha,* meaning five; and *karma,* meaning methods or measures. *Pancha karma* plays a vital role in Ayurvedic medicine, both in health as well as in disease. The five *karmas* are as follows: *Vamana*—emesis; *Virecana*—purgation; *Niruha*—non-oily enema; *Annuvasana*—oily enema; and *Nasya or Sirovirecana*—head evacuation. Some people take *niruha* and *annuvasana* under *vasti* or enema and add the finishing touch to *Pancha karma* by adding *rakta moksana*—blood-letting. Through these five eliminative measures, the toxic matter is evacuated from the body.

The importance of *Pancha karma* in Ayurveda is borne out by the fact that it is applicable to all cases covering a wide range of preventive, curative, and promotive conditions. A common comparison states that just as dyeing is not properly effected if the cloth is not properly washed and cleaned—in the same way—no therapy works well if the purificatory measures are not taken beforehand. It is postulated that the vitiated *doshas* and *malas* of the body need to be eliminated before any specific measure is taken to cure the disease.

Some measures need to be taken before and after the *Pancha karma* therapy is applied. *Purva karma* is the preparatory procedure required to be undertaken before the actual *Pancha karma* therapy is administered. *Paschata karma* advises a special post-therapy dietetic regimen which is designed to restore the digestive and absorptive capacity of the person, thus restoring him to a normal state of health. The *Paschata karma* advised for each type of *Purva karma* and *Pancha karma* is given as Post-procedural precautions.

Pancha karma forms a part of the regimen of preventive medicine, as it is a prophylactic measure in the context of epidemics and pandemics. It is also indicated as a preparatory procedure before surgery, the administration of *rasayana* or *rejuvenation* therapy, and *vajikarana* or the therapy for the promotion of virility and sexual stamina. Thus *Pancha karma* therapy has a direct relevance for both, the healthy as well as the ailing. Each one of the *Pancha karma* procedures have to be applied with due consideration to the particular type of *doshic* disturbances and indications, and contraindications of their use. Therefore, the patient has to be carefully examined, assessed, and prepared before the administration of one or the other procedures.

Purva Karma

Purva karma requires *Snehana* (oleation) and *Swedana* (fomentation).

Snehana Karma: Snehana is the main *Purva karma* procedure. Literally, *snehana* means to oleate or to make smooth. It is a specific treatment for *vatic disorders*. Oily preparations given are *ghee*, oils, and fats.

Indications of *snehana* are sexual exhaustion, anaemia, anxiety, dryness of the body, and senility. It is also given in preparation for *vimana* and *virecana*.

The patient is administered oily preparations within fifteen to thirty minutes after sunrise. The quantity, duration, and the type of preparation is determined beforehand in each case. Certain dietary restrictions are a prerequisite. A liquid diet, well regulated, and taken warm is preferred. One that is too sticky for the body channels or in some way too oleaus, is incompatible.

A close watch should be kept on the patient to ascertain whether the administration of *snehana* is proving effective and adequate. The effectiveness will be indicated by accelerated digestive power, intolerance to fat, loose motions, lightness of the body, smoothness of the body, passage of flatus, visible fat in the stool.

Those who have undergone the treatment are further advised use of warm water; abstinence from sexual activities; sleeping only at night; avoiding anger, anxiety, or loud talk.

Swedana Karma: Swedana is designed to induce sweating by application of heat. There are a number of ways and means to practise this procedure.

Corrhyza, cough, headache, paralysis, constipation, and arthritis are the conditions for which swedana is given.

Generally *vamana* is given on the second day of *swedana,* and *virecana* after three days' interval. If *vasti, nasya, rakta mokasana* are to be given, they may be given immediately after *swedana.*

Disappearance of corrhyza, relief from pain and stiffness, and remission of the disease will illustrate whether *swedana* has been adequately and effectively administered.

The patient should avoid cold water, and take a nap after a light meal.

The Pancha Karmas

Vamana Karma: Vamana karma is an important *pradhana karma* of the *Pancha karma* therapy. Literally, *vamana* means to expel the vitiated *doshas* through the oral route. The expelled material may consist of undigested food, *kapha,* and *pitta. Vamana karma* is a specific therapy for *kaphaja* disorders.

Indications of vamana are nasal discharge, acute fever, cough, tuberculosis, asthma, indigestion, poisoning, nausea, anorexia, obesity, and sore throat.

Vamana should always be preceeded by suitable *purva karmas* in order to mobilize the *doshas.* A variety of *vamana* drugs are used to induce it.

Adequate and effective use of *vamana* is indicated by: maximum elimination of *doshas* with minimal dose; minimisation of the disease; absence of complications; pleasant taste, smell, and colour.

After *vamana* the following should be avoided: loud speech, overeating, continued sitting, too much walking, anger, anxiety, coitus, retention of natural urges.

Virecana Karma: *Virecana karma* is the next major *pradhana karma* included under *Pancha karma* therapy. *Virecana* means to expel the *doshas* through the anal passage. *Virecana* is the specific therapy for *pitta dosa* disorders. *Virecana* expels *pitta* from the *amasaya* (stomach and upper part of the small intestine), which act is not performed by *niruha vasti,* though the latter uses the anal route for elimination.

Virecana is neither stressful nor painful. It is the easiest procedure, usually unaccompanied by any complication. A variety of drugs are used for this purpose.

Indications for *virecana* are fever, skin diseases, piles, splenic disorders, abdominal swellings, headaches, constipation, anorexia, asthma, cough, jaundice, gout, indigestion, gastrointestinal disorders, oedema.

Adequate *virecana* is indicated by a feeling of lightness in the body, lightness in the abdomen and intestines, an increased appetite, and absence of the symptoms of the disease.

After an adequate dose of the purgative has been taken, cleansing of the anal passage follows automatically.

After *virecana karma*, the patient should take plenty of rest and a light diet.

Vasti Karma: *Vasti* is a major procedure among the *Pancha karmas*. The term *vasti* is derived from the fact that the *vasti yantra* or the apparatus used for introducing medicated materials is made up of *vasti* or an animal's urinary bladder. The *vasti* procedure, applied through the anus, may be *niruha vasti* or *annuvasana vasti.*

The *vasti* procedure restores the balance of the *dosas*. It increases weight in emaciated people, decreases weight in the obese, improves vision, prevents ageing, brings back lustre and strength, and healthy longevity. It is specifically for *vatic* disorders.

Indications for *niruha vasti* are retention of flatus, retention of urine, retention of stools, loss of strength, *doshic* deficiency, fever, splenic diseases, abdominal swelling and pain, headache, lumbago, heaviness, oedema, stiffness, gout, piles, dysuria.

Indications for *annuvasana vasti* are coarseness, increased appetite, and an increase of *vata dosha.*

Vasti is of two types; *niruha vasti* which consists of the use of decoction of appropriate drugs; and *annuvasana vasti* which uses oily substances. In many cases, a combination of both these types of *vasti* is given.

Adequate *vasti* is indicated by: proper passage of wind and urine, a proper balance of *doshas,* a feeling of lightness in the body, a pleasant feeling, increased appetite and strength.

A light diet should be taken after *vasti.* The following activities should be avoided after *vasti:* sitting for a long duration, standing for a long duration, excessive talking, travelling, sleeping during the day, coitus, sexual relationship, anxiety, anger, untimely meals, an incompatible diet.

Sirovirecana Karma: *Sirovirecana or Nasya* is generally the last step in the *pradhana karma* of the *Pancha karma* therapy. *Nasya* is a term applied for medicines or medicated oils administered through the nasal passage. *Nasya karma* is considered the best and the most specific procedure for diseases of the head (*siro*). The nasal passage is considered to be the portal of the head, and, accordingly, all drugs and measures introduced through the nose spread throughout the head and its constituent parts, and influence all the *doshas* and the diseases situated in these parts.

Nasya karma is said to prevent diseases of the eyes, ears, and nose; promote healthy hair; improve the voice; delay ageing; and bestow a pleasant oral smell.

A stiff neck, stiff jaw, chronic corrhyza, tonsillitis, cataract, headache, earache, shoulder ache, tooth ache, hoarseness of voice, stammering, alteration of voice are indications for the use of *sirovirecana.*

The following four types of *nasya* procedures may be administered:

Navana nasya. It is administered by instilling the drops of a medicated oil in the nose.

Auapida nasya. It is administered by instilling the juice (extract) of a drug through the nasal passages.

Dhamapana or Pradhamana nasya. It is administered by inhaling the fine powder of drugs in the nasal passages with the help of a *nadi-yantra*.

Dhuma nasya. It is administered by inhaling medicated fumes through the nasal passages and eliminating them through the oral route.

Long lists of drugs that can be taken as *nasya* are given in ancient Ayurvedic texts.

During the *nasya* procedure, the head should not be excessively flexed or bent, and the patient should be supine. He should avoid speech, anger, laughing, swallowing, and clearing his throat.

Adequate *nasya* is indicated by lightness of the body, good sleep, lightness of the head, and a feeling of pleasure.

After the *nasya* procedure, the patient should avoid cold water, oils and *ghee*, alcohol, and a headbath. Inhalation of dust and fumes should be avoided.

Note: Some Ayurvedic texts, particularly *Susruta Samhita,* include *rakta moksana* (blood-letting) as one of the *Pancha karmas*. They consider the two types of *vasti* as one, and thus stick to the stipulated number of five *karmas*.

Keraliya Pancha Karma

A simplified form of the *Pancha karma* therapy has been practised in Kerala for a long time. This practice, which is very different to the classical *Pancha karma* is popularly known as *Keraliya Pancha karma*. The five major components of Keraliya *Pancha karma* are as follows:

1. *Dhara karma*
2. *Kaya seka*
3. *Pinda sweda*
4. *Anna lepa*
5. *Siro lepa*

Dhara Karma: A liquid medicament like medicated oil, milk, *ghee, takra, or kwatha* (decoction of drugs) is placed in a pot with a thin hole at the bottom. The pot is hung at an appropriate height, and the liquid is allowed to trickle slowly through the pot on to the forehead of the patient, lying below on a *droni* (wooden plank). In this procedure, the medicated liquid is selected in consideration of the nature of illness, and the constitution and strength of the patient. This procedure has been found to be very effective in patients suffering from mental diseases, and diseases of the, eye, ear, nose, and throat. It has also been found effective for diseases like facial palsy, insomnia, and diminished memory.

***Kaya Seka* or *Sarvanga Sencana*:** Medicated liquid such as an oil is poured all over the body of the patient using the previous procedure of *dhara karma.* The material is poured from a particular height, and a simultaneous massage is also done. This procedure provides strength to the tissues. The lustre and beauty of the body is enhanced; the sense organs become clear; and longevity is achieved. This procedure helps regeneration and rejuvenation of the body, and is especially good in the management of *vatika* diseases.

Kaya seka provides simultaneous *snehana* and *swedana.* It is administered for one hour and increased upto one-and-a-half hours for fourteen days or twenty-one days. At the end of the procedure, the patient is asked to sit down, and his shoulders and the neck are vigorously massaged. Then the patient is given a bath. At the same time, the oils and medicaments remaining on the body of the patient are removed by rubbing with a towel.

Pinda Sweda: A bolus of *payasam* (paste), made up of new coarse rice *(sastika sali)* cooked in milk, is used for fomenting or massage of the body. Prior to the actual *pinda sweda* procedure, it is essential to do adequate *snehana* by applying oil all over the body. After that the body should be fomented with lukewarm medicated paste encapsulated in a piece of cloth. After a few rounds of fomentation with the wrapped bolus, the cloth is opened, and the entire body is systematically massaged by rubbing the warm paste all over.

The entire process can be ended with a warm water bath, followed by rest at room temperature.

Swedana with *pinda* is done for one hour and forty-five minutes. Then the body is wiped with an oily piece of cloth. Following this, a medicated oil bath is given which, in turn, is followed by a bath with lukewarm water. This therapy is given daily or on alternate days. Depending upon the nature of the disease, the therapy is continued for 7, 11, 14, 21, or 28 days.

Pinda sweda relieves tiredness, depression, drowsiness, and insomnia. It promotes appetite. The stiffness of the joints disappears.

A successfully employed *pinda sweda* is believed to help, to a great extent, patients suffering from different neuromuscular disorders and systemic diseases.

Anna Lepa: Specially processed and medicated *anna* (cereal) is used for applying on the body in some conditions when *pinda sweda* does not work.

The procedure of preparation of *anna lepa dravya* (medicated cereal paste) is the same as is used for preparing the *pinda sweda dravya.*

The patient is asked to lie down in a *droni.* Lukewarm *lepa* is applied all over the body except the head. *Anna lepa* therapy is administered in several body postures as is the case for *pinda* therapy. It is continued for one to one-and-a-half hours. When the *lepa* becomes cold, it is made warm. After that the *lepa* is removed. It iṣ followed by *snehana* and then, a warm water wash.

Siro Lepa: Siro lepa is indicated in cases of mental and brain disorders where the paste of traditionally known drugs is applied on the head of the patient.

In *Keraliya Pancha karma,* the selection of drugs for preparing *dhara, lepa, or pinda* is done by taking into consideration the nature of the disease to be treated. Therefore medicaments are specific for that disease, whether applied externally or given internally. These procedures render the channels of the body free from stagnation, making the sticky contents mobile, and directing them in an appropriate direction. This automatically leads to elimination or excretion of the *doshas*, even without applying the classical *sodhana* or purificatory measures. Keraliya physicians advocate *Pancha karma* to be administered preferably in the rainy season, as this is the time when the *vata dosha* gets disturbed and needs to be curbed.

It is essential that for one week prior to the *Pancha karma,* the patient is kept under observation,during which period, the procedure best suited for the patient is decided upon. After the therapy, a medicated lukewarm water bath is recommended, accompanied by a light diet. Excessive physical and mental exertion should be avoided, as also sexual intercourse.

In the chapters on diseases that follow, besides the other modes of treatment recommended in the text, the *Pancha karma* therapy may be applied wherever indicated.

Fevers

नवज्वरे दिवारव्वपनरनानाभ्यडगचमैथुनम् ।
क्रोधप्रवातव्यायामान् कषायांश्रच विवर्जयेत् ॥

When fever strikes, the patient should not be permitted to sleep during the day, bathe, apply oil on the body, have sexual intercourse, or get angry. Going out in the open where the winds blow strongly, taking exercise, and eating of astringent substances should also be prohibited.

CHARAKA SAMHITA

FEVER MAY be defined as an increase in body temperature to above normal. The term has a very wide application, as fever is one of the most common accompaniments of diseases in general, and infections in particular. In many cases fever must be regarded as secondary to and symptomatic of a diseased state with which it is associated.

The average temperature of the healthy body ranges between 36.9° and 37.5°C or 98.4° and 99.5°F and is liable to slight variations from such causes as the ingestion of food, the amount of exercise undertaken, and the temperature of the surrounding atmosphere. The body experiences its lowest temperature between 1.30 a.m. and 7 a.m. and the highest between 4 p.m. and 9 p.m.

If the fever rises to 41.1°C or 106°F, the term *hyperpyrexia* is applied. Hyperpyrexia is a signal of danger for the patient. If the fever exceeds 41.7°C or 42.2°C for any length of time, death almost always ensues. Occasionally, the temperature may rise as high as 43.3°C to 44.5°C prior to death. The onset of the fever may be associated with a rigor or shivering, pain in the back, headache, thirst, and great lassitude. These symptoms, however, vary according to the type of fever. For example, a cardinal symptom of typhoid or enteric fever is a slow pulse in spite of a high temperature, whereas, in an infection of the urinary tract, the pulse is extremely rapid as compared to the temperature of the body.

Even though fever is generally translated as *jwara*, the connotation of the term *jwara* in Ayurveda is slightly different. It includes not only the rise in body temperature, but also the troubles that afflict the mind, the five special sense organs, and the body. *Dehendriya Manastapi* is, therefore, the appropriate description of fever in Ayurveda.

Varieties of Fever

Charaka has categorized fever into several varieties depending upon the vitiation of the three *doshas,* namely, *vata*, *pitta,* and *kapha;* the change of climate or seasons; the vitiation of the vital fluid blood; and other supplementary reasons. Modern medicine associates fevers with the following diseases: typhoid, meningitis, dengue fever, diphtheria, sandfly fever, yellow fever, mumps, rheumatic fever, heat exhaustion and heat stroke, measles, bulbous eruptions, erysipelas, hectic fever, malaria, black-water fever, *kala-azar*, filaria.[1]

Fevers associated with different diseases are discussed under their related systems. For example: Influenza, pneumonia, and tuberculosis are discussed under Diseases of the Respiratory Organs, and so on.

Fevers are also classified according to their severity and duration. Ayurvedic teachers have specified the role of the *Pancha karmas* or five cleansing procedures (as described in Chapter 5) for the various fevers and the stages at which they come to the notice of the physician. In some fevers, the patient may have to fast or be kept on liquids, whereas in others, soft foods may be permitted. In yet others, where there is no

---

1. It would be relevant here to point out that the once dreaded disease, smallpox, has been eradicated all over the world.

involvement of the digestive system, this type of dietary restriction is not needed.

Typhoid Fever *(Aantrik Jwara)*

Typhoid or enteric fever, so named due to the involvement of the intestines, is one of the more difficult fevers to deal with, and has a tendency to emaciate the patient, if not checked in time. It has an insidious onset; there may be ulceration of the bowels or ulceration of the skin through eruptions. Typhoid fever has a tendency to relapse.

Causes and Symptoms: According to modern medicine, a bacillus, *Salmonella typhi*, is the cause of the disease. The fever comes on gradually, allowing the victim to move about normally for some days after the onset. The most marked symptoms are headache, lassitude, and discomfort. These are accompanied by insomnia and feverishness, particularly, at night. In the beginning, the temperature is slightly higher than normal in the morning, and even higher in the evening. The fever increases gradually to the highest point on the eighth day. The malady may continue for as long as three weeks or even twenty-eight days. Relapses are not uncommon and have to be guarded against. A marked feature of typhoid is that the pulse rate does not rise corresponding to the body temperature as happens in other fevers. Of course, in protracted cases where there is extensive ulceration of the intestines, the pulse may become weak and rapid. Right from the start, abdominal symptoms such as distension of the abdomen, and pain and gurgling sounds when light pressure is exerted on the lower abdomen, can be observed. Diarrhoea is a frequent, but by no means, a constant symptom.

If ulceration of the bowels is not treated in time, they may get perforated; this is almost, always, a fatal symptom. According to Ayurveda, typhoid is the result of vitiation of all the three *doshas* in the body.

43

Medicines and Prescriptions:

FIRST WEEK:

1. *Mrigshringa Bhasma; Muktashukti Bhasma.*

120 mg each of *Mrigshringa Bhasma* and *Muktashukti Bhasma* to be given thrice daily with honey.

2. *Khub Kalan.*

A decoction of 12 gm of *Khub Kalan* and 10 gm of dried grapes, with one litre of water, boiled down to about one-third, should be given along with the above medicines.

SECOND WEEK:

1. *Kasturibhairava; Muktashukti Bhasma.*

120 mg of *Kasturibhairava* and 12 mg of *Muktashukti Bhasma* to be taken twice daily with honey.

2. *Jwararyabhra; Saubhagya Vati.*

120 mg of *Jwararyabhra* and 240 mg of *Saubhagya Vati* to be taken twice daily with juice of fresh ginger.

THIRD WEEK:

1. *Vasantamalati; Pravala Bhasma; Amritasatva.*

120 mg of *Vasantamalati*, 120 mg of *Pravala Bhasma*, and 120 mg of *Amritasatva* to be taken in the morning and evening with honey.

2. *Sarvajwaralauha; Pippali Churna.*

240 mg of *Sarvajwaralauha* and 240 mg of *Pippali Churna* to be taken in the morning and evening with honey.

FOURTH WEEK:

1. *Vasantamalati; Navayasa Churna; Sitopaladi.*

120 mg of *Vasantamalati*, 240 mg of *Navayasa Churna*, 1.5 gm of *Sitopaladi* to be taken morning and evening with honey.

44

2. *Vishmushtayasava;* *Lauhasava;* *Amritarishta.*	5 ml of *Vishmushtayasava*, 10 ml of *Lauhasava*, and 10 ml of *Amritarishta* to be taken twice daily after meals.

In addition, *Mahalakshadi* oil should be used for massage of the body.

Diet and Other Regimen: During an attack of typhoid, diet is of the utmost importance because of the involvement of the intestines. Soft liquid foods, particularly, milk and fruit juices are the best. All substances which are likely to irritate the digestive processes should be avoided. The main consideration is that there should not be any burden on the digestive system, nor should constipation be allowed to develop.

Since the disease causes a lot of weakness, bedrest during the disease and for about a week afterwards is recommended. A glycerine suppository may be resorted to in cases of constipation.

Meningitis *(Mastishka Shoth)*

Meningitis is the inflammation of the membranes of the brain. It may occur independently, or may be the result of such diseases as tuberculosis. In either case, the brain and, sometimes, the spinal coverings are involved.

Causes and Symptoms: Except in the case of pneumococcal or tuberculous meningitis, the onset of meningitis is sudden, the temperature rising from 39° to 41.1°C. Vomiting, headache, and shivering appear first, followed by stiffness of the neck. Convulsions are common among children. The patient may fall down suddenly and go into convulsions, or he may go to bed and be found unconscious the following morning. The meningitis patient suffers from irritability, insomnia, and even delirium. His body is tender to touch. The limbs are so stiff that the pressing of the lower limbs on the abdomen with the knees straight becomes impossible. Sometimes red spots appear on the patient's skin. This condition is called 'spotted fever'. If unchecked, cardiac failure may occur within a week, resulting in death. Meningitis or cerebro-spinal fever may last from two to four days, or stretch over some months. If the patient survives the first week, chances of recovery are favourable.

Medicines and Prescriptions: The following medicines may be taken in consultation with a physician:

1. *Vata Chintamani; Kasturi Bhairava; Krishna Chaturmukha.*

120 mg each of *Vata Chintamani, Kasturi Bhairava,* and *Krishna Chaturmukha* to be taken thrice daily.

2. *Siddha Makaradhwaja; Saubhagya Vati.*

120 mg of *Siddha Makaradhwaja* and 240 mg of *Saubhagya Vati* to be taken twice daily with juice of fresh ginger.

In addition to the above medicines, *Mahavishagarbha Taila* should be used for massaging the back, particularly the spinal region. Diuretics (medicines increasing the flow of urine) should be taken to help the patient to relieve cerebral oedema, if present.

Diet and Other Regimen: When the patient is conscious, a liquid diet may be given orally, care being taken that there is no aspiration of food into the lungs.

During the disease, if weakness of any part of the body develops, physiotherapy is called for.

Dengue Fever *(Dandak Jwara)*

Dengue fever, also called Dandy fever, Three-day fever (due to its duration), and Breakbone fever, is a disease of the tropical and sub-tropical region.

Causes and Symptoms: Dengue fever is transmitted by infected mosquitoes. Its onset is sudden and it is characterised by swelling and pains in the joints and muscles. Eruptions may also appear on various parts of the body along with the above symptoms. The throat is sore and the eyes, watery. The symptoms gradually pass off in three days, leaving the patient very weak. Relapses occur frequently causing the disease to

46

last for as long as one month. Dengue fever, however, is not a fatal disease.

The temperature pattern in this fever shows a sudden rise, followed by a relative fall, and then a sudden fall again. That is why the temperature in dengue fever is called a 'saddleback' type temperature.

One should remember that over-medication in dengue fever is likely to lead to further complications. A mild attack of the fever may pass off without having to administer any medicine.

Medicines & Prescriptions: *Hinguleshwar*—120 mg, and 360 mg of *Shunthi Churna* should be taken four times daily with hot water. In case the temperature goes beyond 40°C, cold compresses should be applied.

Diet and Other Regimen: The dietary restrictions are the same as in the case of other fevers. The patient should be kept on a liquid diet, preferably milk and fruit juices. Substances that are likely to irritate the digestive organs should be avoided.

Since the disease causes aches and pains all over the body, particularly in the backbone, massage and fomentation with a hot water bottle will provide relief. Mild laxatives are recommended in case there is constipation.

Diphtheria *(Rohini)*

Diphtheria, which is a bacterial infection caused by *Corynebacterium diptheriae,* is an acute infectious disease, accompanied by a membranous exudation on a mucous surface—generally on the tonsils, and back of the throat or pharynx. Toxins in the exudation are likely to harm the heart muscle and the nerves.

Causes and Symptoms: Diphtheria is predominantly a disease of autumn and winter, and although it affects all ages, it is more common in childhood. It begins as an inflammation of the throat. Next, a membrane develops over the throat, choking the patient. If this membrane extends into the air passage, the patient experiences asphyxia (inability to breathe). It is rare among infants upto the age of six months. According to Ayurveda, diphtheria is the result of the vitiation of the *kapha.*

47

The toxin of diphtheria has a special predilection for the heart as it attacks it vehemently, resulting in its failure. The temperature in this disease rarely rises beyond 39.4° C, but the pulse is weak and rapid, and the countenance pale. The swelling of the glands in the neck increases rapidly, leading to blood poisoning.

Medicines & Prescriptions:

1. *Shuddha Visha; Kasturi Bhairava; Shringa Bhasma; Kalaka Churna.*

   20 mg of *Shuddha Visha,* 30 mg each of *Kasturi Bhairava* and *Shringa Bhasma,* 240 mg of *Kalaka Churna* to be taken every three hours till relief is noticed.

2. *Shuddha Tankan; Yavakshara; Katphaladi Churna.*

   260 mg of *Shuddha Tankan,* 750 mg of *Yavakshara,* 4 gm of *Katphaladi Churna* to be mixed with honey and juice of ginger, and used as a linctus.

The course of the disease is extremely rapid. If proper medication is not given in time, there is little hope for survival of the patient. Sometimes surgical help has to be sought. Normally the surgeons make a supplementary air passage to let the patient breathe, and, in the meantime, medication is given.

Allopathy has developed a serum which, if injected in childhood, gives lifelong immunity against the disease. Normally, it is a part of the triple antigen which is administered to infants.

Diet and Other Regimen: The patient may be put on a liquid diet. A mouthwash after each meal is recommended.

Sandfly Fever *(Marumakshika Jwara)*

Sandfly fever, also known as Three-day fever (due to its duration) is a short, sharp fever. It is common at the junction of the seasons, and is endemic to the northern regions of India, particularly Punjab, Delhi, Western U.P., and Madhya Pradesh.

Causes and Symptoms: Sandfly fever is caused by the sandfly—a small, hair midge called *Phlebotomus papatasi*, which ordinarily infests refuse heaps.

The cardinal symptoms of the disease are: headache, feverishness, a flushed face, general sensations which an influenza patient has, bloodshot eyes, but no catarrh. The temperature goes upto 40°C and returns to normal after three days; sometimes, there may be a relapse. The pulse is weak and thready.

Medicines & Prescriptions: *Hinguleshwar—120 mg,* 180 mg of *Godanti Bhasma,* and 240 mg of *Amritasatva* should be taken four times a day with honey.

Diet and Other Regimen: As no digestive disorders accompany this fever, the dietary restrictions are a little relaxed. Even so, soft and easily-digestible foods are recommended.

The patient must ensure that he gets proper rest, and see that his bowels function normally. In case of constipation, a suppository or a mild laxative is recommended.

Mumps *(Karnamulaka Jwara)*

Mumps is an infectious disease caused by a virus. It occurs frequently in an epidemic form in winter or spring, and mostly affects children. If it occurs in later life, it usually leads to other complications such as orchitis (inflammation of the testicles), resulting in atrophy of the testicles, and later, sterility among males.

Causes and Symptoms: The first signs are fatigue, slight feverishness, and a sore throat which may precede the swelling of the parotid gland, which is situated in front of and below the ear. Facial pain and temperature upto 40°C follow, and inflammation spreads to the glands below the jaw. After four or five days, both the swelling and the temperature subside. If the disease attacks adults (fortunately, it seldom does), there may be swelling of the testicles in males, and the ovaries among females.

49

Medicines & Prescriptions:

1. *Mrigshringa Bhasma; Sanjivani.*	10 mg of *Mrigshringa Bhasma* and 120 mg of *Sanjivani* to be taken with warm water or juice of ginger four times a day.
2. *Ashwakanchuki.*	120 to 240 mg to be given at night with warm water.

Home Remedies: The affected part may be covered with a poultice consisting of *Nalukakepa* or *Dashangalepa* and *ghee.* It must be covered with a cotton or woollen cloth to keep it warm.

Diet and Other Regimen: Soft, liquid foods are recommended. As a matter of fact, they are the only foods that the patient can take since the inflammation of the glands under the jaw makes swallowing of any solid substances painful.

Hot fomentation over the swollen glands is not recommended. The patient may keep a lozenge or a piece of candy in his mouth to facilitate salivation. This will bring down the swelling faster.

Rheumatic Fever *(Aamavata Jwara)*

Rheumatic fever is a general disorder accompanied by pain in the joints, feverishness, and copious perspiration. The disease is one to which children and adolescents are more prone; it is generally not evidenced among people over thirty years of age. If the disease attacks an individual upto the age of eighteen, proper care and medication can control the disease. The disease has a tendency to spread in an erratic manner, and involves the smooth membranes of the body, particularly, the heart.

Causes and Symptoms: An attack of rheumatic fever generally begins with a chill, followed by fever. It is accompanied by a feeling of stiffness or pain in one or more joints, usually of the knees, ankles, wrists, or shoulders. With the passage of time, the pain becomes really severe. The patient's face becomes flushed and his whole body is bathed in perspiration. The temperature is usually 39.4°C, the pulse rapid but strong, the tongue coated. The patient also suffers from excessive thirst, loss of appetite, and constipation. The attack lasts for a few days if there is no relapse.If the disease is not controlled, certain complications may develop. Inflammation of the outer membrane, the inner membrane, and the muscle of the heart may develop. The risk of cardiac complications is greater among patients of tender age since their joints are small and their swelling may sometimes be overlooked. Another serious complication which is noticed in some cases is hyperpyrexia (high fever), ranging from 41.1°C to 42.2°C.

Medicines & Prescriptions:

1. *Hinguleshwar; Aamavatari Rasa; Saubhagya Vati.* — 120 mg of *Hinguleshwar,* with 240 mg each of *Aamavatari Rasa* and *Saubhagya Vati* to be administered thrice daily with warm water.

2. *Vishveshwara Rasa; Shringa Bhasma; Yavakshara; Hritpatri (digitalis).* — 120 mg each of *Vishveshwara Rasa* and *Shringa Bhasma;* 240 mg each of *Yavakshara* and *Hritpatri*—all four medicines to be given twice daily with honey.

Home Remedies: A hot compress of sand or salt put in a bag and heated over a hot plate, should be applied to the swollen joints. Leaves of *amarbel* or *dhatura* heated over a hot plate may be applied to the affected joints as a poultice.

Diet and Other Regimen: As a dietary supplement, *Panchkol-shruta* milk may be given thrice daily in quantities of upto 180 ml. Soft and warm foods, and substances such as bitter gourd which contain acrid components, are recommended.

Complete rest is advised for patients of rheumatic fever, and diuretics should be administered in appropriate cases. Constipation should be treated with laxatives.

Heat Exhaustion and Heat Stroke

(Aanshughata Jwara and Anshughata Sannipata)

Heat exhaustion and heat stroke are diseases common to tropical climates.

Causes and Symptoms: In India these disorders strike people in summer when the temperature rises; those living or moving about in open air without proper clothing or precautions are more susceptible than others. Profuse sweating due to atmospheric heat leads to severe loss of vital salts in the body, and a condition known as heat exhaustion develops, in which the patient feels faint and may even fall unconscious. Another reason for heat exhaustion is dehydration, which may also result in unconsciousness.

Heat exhaustion is a precursor to heat stroke. The latter is characterised by high fever, absence of sweating, thirst, a rapid pulse, confusion, and, sometimes, loss of consciousness.

The fever of heat stroke comes on suddenly, with the temperature rising from 41.1°C to 42.2°C. Anal temperature sometimes touches 44.5°C. Severe ache in the body, particularly in the head, is followed by confusion, cramps, a sense of impending doom, and loss of consciousness. If immediate steps are not taken, the patient may die of dyspnoea (difficulty in breathing).

Heat Exhaustion

- Sweaty, pale, cool skin
- No fever
- Pupils
- weakness

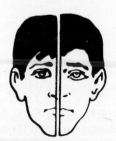

Heat Stroke

- Dry, red hot skin
- High fever
- The person is very ill or unconscious

**Differences Between
Heat Exhaustion and Heat Stroke**

Home Remedies: In case the temperature reaches 40°C and appears to rise further, immediate steps should be taken. The patient must be divested of all his clothes and his body wrapped in a sheet soaked in iced water. Alternatively, he should be made to lie down under a shower bath and his body cooled till the temperature returns to 38.9°C When the temperature starts falling and the pulse shows signs of weakness, 50 to 75 ml of *Mritsanjivani Sura* should be given.

Medicines & Prescriptions:

1. *Ratneshwar Rasa; Chandandi Churna.*	120 mg of *Ratneshwar Rasa* and 240 mg of *Chandandi Churna* to be taken thrice daily with *Triphala* water.
2. *Mahashishir Panak.*	*Mahashishir Panak* should be given to the patient in 10 ml doses every half an hour.

Diet and Other Regimen: The adage 'Prevention is better than cure', applies more to heat stroke than to any other malady. One should take care to take water at frequent intervals during summer. A little salt may be added to it before one goes outdoors in the summer sun. This will maintain the balance of the vital salts in the body. *Panna* (soup made of raw mangoes), taken once during the day, helps in preventing heat stroke. Drinking liquids, even if one does not feel thirsty, is essential in summer. This prevents the body fluids from falling below the minimum levels due to excessive sweat and perspiration.

The patient may be kept on a normal diet depending on his appetite which is affected in some cases of fever. Hard-to-digest foods should be avoided.

Whenever one goes out in summer, the head and the back of the neck should be covered with a thick cloth. During heat exhaustion or a heat stroke, the use of purgatives should be avoided.

Chickenpox *(Laghu Masurika)*

Chickenpox is an acute contagious disease, common to children, particularly between the ages of one to ten years. Though it has a superficial resemblance to smallpox, it is entirely a different disease and less severe.

Causes and Symptoms: Caused by a virus, the disease starts with slight feverishness, and pain in the back and legs. There may be a feeling of chill, and with twenty-four hours of its onset, small red pappules appear on the back and chest, and, sometimes, on the forehead too. The pimples turn into vesicles (filled with a clear liquid), but within a day or two, they either suppurate or shrivel up with a brown crust appearing on them. The eruptions last several days.

Medicines & Prescriptions: Even without medication, chickenpox will pass off without any ill effects in about a week. In adults, however, though the disease strikes infrequently, it may cause extreme weakness and prostration.

FIRST WEEK:

1. *Swarnamakshika Bhasma.*	120 mg of *Swarnamaksnika Bhasma* to be taken morning and evening with decoction of *Kanchnar tree bark.*
2. *Eladyarishta.*	20 ml of *Eladyarishta* to be taken after meals with water.

SECOND WEEK:

1. *Indukala Vatika.*	120 mg of *Indukala Vatika* to be taken morning and evening.
2. *Haridra Churna.*	1 gm of *Haridra Churna* to be taken with juice of bitter gourd leaves at noon and night.

Diet and Other Regimen: The patient may be kept on a normal diet depending upon his appetite which is affected in some cases of fever. Hard-to digest-foods should be avoided.

Purgatives should be avoided.

Measles *(Romantika)*

Measles is an acute, infectious disease which strikes mostly children. The more tender the age, the better is the ability to bear the troubles that measles brings. It is generally believed that one attack of the disease provides immunity against a second attack. But that is the general rule to which many exceptions have been noticed. The second attack generally comes if the first one has been of a very mild nature. Like chickenpox, measles is contagious, and the sufferer should be segregated at the first onset of the symptoms.

Causes and Symptoms: Ayurveda believes that measles is the result of vitiation of both *kapha* and *pitta*. In the beginning, there is acute catarrh, followed by sneezing, a watery discharge, and, sometimes, bleeding from the nose. There is a dry cough and hoarseness of voice. The temperature goes up to 40°C and the pulse is rapid. Headache, thirst, and restlessness are also present. The temperature recedes on the third day, and on the fourth day, the characteristic rash of measles appears. The rash is first noticed on the brow, cheeks, chin, behind the ears, and on the neck. It consists of small spots of a dusky red or crimson colour, slightly elevated above the surface of the skin. The face acquires a swollen and bloated appearance. Sometimes the rash also appears in the mouth and the throat. It continues for two or three days and then subsides. A slight peeling of the skin may take place during convalescence. The appearance of the rash should be taken as a sign of the start of the recovery.

In certain rare cases, measles may occur in a very severe or malignant form, giving rise to complications. If the bronchial tubes or the lungs are involved, the result may be fatal. Almost all fatal cases are the result of involvement of the lungs or the bronchi.

Home Remedies: The first thing to be done when the disease is suspected to be measles, is to clothe the patient in warm garments. Hot water and other liquids should be given to encourage the rash to appear. One of the grandmother's nostrums is to give the child raisins to eat. Powdered liquorice

55

root may be given with honey. A powder of equal parts of tamarind seeds and turmeric may be given in doses of 350 to 425 mg thrice daily.

Medicines & Prescriptions: Before the rash appears, the following medicines should be administered: 120 mg each of *Swarnamakshika Bhasma, Kasturi Bhairava, Shringa Bhasma;* and 240 mg of *Saubhagya Vati*—all to be taken four times daily with juice of bitter gourd and honey.

Unless accompanied by morbid complications, measles will cure automatically. But the most important precaution to be taken is not to suppress the fever of measles as that is likely to lead to a more virulent attack.

Diet and Other Regimen: The patient may be given a normal diet depending upon his appetite, but-hard-to digest foods, fatty substances, and those which are likely to lead to constipation should be avoided.

The patient should not be exposed to draughts, and should be advised to lie down in a soft bed in a slightly darkened room. He should be segregated.

Bulbous Eruptions *(Visphotaka Jwara)*

There is another type of fever—*Visphotaka Jwara*—the one which accompanies eruptions, particularly bulbous eruptions. Bulbous eruptions have been treated by the author of the *Bhaishajaratnavali* as a sign of smallpox, but Sushruta differentiated between the two, calling the former a minor disease.

Causes and Symptoms: Ayurveda states that bulbous eruptions are due to the vitiation of the *pitta* and the blood. Sushruta categorised these eruptions into seven classes: three caused by vitiation of any of the three *doshas* of the body; three caused by the interaction of the *doshas;* and one caused by the vitiation of all the three *doshas* together.

Medicines & Prescriptions: *Chandanadi Lauha*—240 mg, along with 120 mg each of *Shuddha Gandhaka* and *Pravala Pishti*, should be taken thrice daily with candy (*mishri*).

Diet and Other Regimen: No diet restrictions are necessary and a normal diet is advised. However, hard-to-digest foods should be avoided.

Purgatives should be avoided.

Erysipelas *(Visarpa)*

Erysipelas is a disease of the skin and subcutaneous tissue. It is a disease characterised by diffused inflammation of the skin or of the subcutaneous cellular tissue, attended with fever. When the disease is in a mild form, the skin becomes red, hard, and thick. Small vesicles appear on it. The redness tends to spread to the neighbouring areas of the skin and the whole body may be involved in the inflammatory process. If the subcutaneous tissue is involved, pus may form under the skin.

Causes and Symptoms: Erysipelas of the face begins with symptoms of general illness. The patient feels languid, drowsy, and sick. There is frequent shivering, and later, fever. The temperature may rise to 40°C or 40.6°C, and inflammation may appear on the face, beginning with the tip of the nose. If the inflammation is not controlled in time and spreads to the throat, the wind pipe may become involved, leading to fatal results. If the inflammation attacks the membranes of the brain, the result is almost always fatal.

Ayurveda believes erysipelas to be the result of the vitiation of all the three *doshas*. It is categorised according to the *dosha* involved. It is of seven types, but Sushruta has mentioned five varieties: three born of the vitiation of any of the three *doshas*; one born of more than one *dosha;* and another caused by injury.

The various varieties of erysipelas and its symptoms differ according to the *dosha* involved, but most of the symptoms common to all the varieties are: inflammation of the skin and the cellular tissues underneath the epidermis; fever and other symptoms present in a fever. When the disease is in a mild form, there is only redness of the skin.

Home Remedies: The inflamed skin should be treated with *Dashangalepa* to which cow's ghee should be added. It should be rubbed gently over the affected part of the skin.

The patient may be bled for quick results, but that should be done under the supervision of an expert in the techniques of blood-letting. Any excessive loss of blood could pose a danger to the life of the patient.

Medicines and Prescriptions:

1. *Kalagnirudra Rasa; Pippali Churna.*	120 mg each of *Kalagnirudra Rasa* and *Pippali Churna* to be given thrice daily with honey.
2. *Nimbadi Quath.*	50 ml to be given once in the morning.

Diet and Other Regimen: The dietary regimen is the same as in the case of other fevers.

The patient must avoid a cold bath and exposure to cold wind as that is likely to aggravate his condition.

Hectic Fever *(Pralepaka Jwara)*

Hectic fever is known as *Pralepaka Jwara* in Ayurveda.

Causes and Symptoms: Hectic fever may occur in certain severe forms of tuberculosis or septicemia. It is mild in intensity and appears in the evening. It ranges between 39°C and 40°C and falls to normal at night, and, sometimes, below normal. There is also profuse sweating accompanied by extreme weakness and even prostration.

Medicines & Prescriptions: If the fever is a symptom of tuberculosis, the following prescription should be tried:

Swarna Vasantamalati; Pravala Bhasma; Yakshamari Lauha; Sitopaladi.	120 mg each of *Swarna Vasantamalati* and *Pravala Bhasma*, 240 mg of *Yakshamari Lauha* and 1 gm of *Sitopaladi* to be given with honey thrice daily.

If attendant upon septicaemia, the fever can be controlled by the administration of the following prescription:

Shri Jaimangala Rasa;	60 mg of
Sanjivani;	*Shri Jaimangala Rasa,*
Shringa Bhasma.	and 120 mg each of *Sanjivani* and *Shringa Bhasma* to be given thrice daily with honey.

Diet and Other Regimen: The patient may be given a normal diet depending upon his appetite, but hard-to-digest foods, fatty substances, and those which are likely to lead to constipation should be avoided.

The patient should not be exposed to draughts.

Malaria *(Vishama Jwara)*

Malaria, which is derived from the Italian *mala aria*—bad air—is also known as ague, paludism, jungle fever, marsh fever, and periodic fever. Malaria is also the main variety of 'intermittent fever' or *Vishama* which has a tendency to return or recur after it subsided.

Causes and Symptoms: Malaria, as a disease, has been known since ancient times, but it was only in 1898 when it was conclusively proved that the Anopheles mosquito transmits the disease.

Malaria is found all over the world, but is endemic in tropical climates where there are marshes or pools of stagnant water, rank vegetation, and a poorly-fed population.

An interesting fact is that it is the female mosquito that bites the prospective malarial patient. The male mosquito does not carry the parasites which cause the disease. The parasites transmitted by the female mosquito enter the blood stream and reach the liver where they mature and multiply. From there, they are released into the blood stream.

Whatever may be the causative organism, the susceptibility to disease is also another factor. If that were not so, all persons exposed to mosquitoes of the malarial variety would suffer from malaria. According to Ayurveda, this susceptibility increases or decreases according to the vitiation of the three *doshas* of the body. *Acharyas* have categorised malaria according to the predominant *dosha,* whose vitiation leads to an attack of malaria.

For a day or two before the actual fever sets in, there may be headache, vague pain in the body and the limbs, accompanied by a feeling of chill, and a slight rise of temperature. An acute malarial attack has three stages: the cold stage, the hot stage, and the sweating stage. The cold stage begins with a feeling of intense chill even in the hottest weather. In spite of the chill the temperature keeps rising. The hot stage comes on as the temperature of the body rises. It begins with hot flushes, which lengthen till the body feels burning hot, the fever rising to 40.6° or 41.1°C. The patient also experiences headache, dizziness, pain throughout the body, and even delirium. This stage may last for hours. After the fever has reached its highest point, the third stage begins. It starts with profuse sweating and a gradual lowering of the body temperature. As the temperature falls, the dizziness, headaches, and pain in the body recede, and the patient feels relieved though weakness persists.

Types of Malaria: Depending upon the parasite which causes it, malaria can be of three types:
quartan fever
tertian fever
malignant tertian malaria

In **quartan fever,** there is an intermission of two days before the next attack, that is, if the first attack is on the first day of the month, the succeeding attacks will be on the 4th, 7th, and 10th days. In **tertian fever,** the attacks occur on alternate days. **Malignant tertian fever** refers to tertian fever in a severe form. In **aestivo-autumnal** fever (relating to autumn, as the name suggests), each attack may last for considerably more than one day and the next attack may come immediately thereafter. The patient is then in a state of fever known as **subtertian** fever. If the infection is severe, malarial fever may occur everyday.

As a rule, after passing through an ague, patients feel completely recovered till the next attack is due, but the fever may not subside. For example, hyperpyrexia (very high fever) may develop and the temperature may continue to rise till death intervenes. The second stage——the hot stage—may continue, without giving way to the third or the sweating stage, and the patient may lose consciousness. If the malarial parasites block the small blood vessels of the brain, cerebral malaria, which is very serious, may develop. This is in most cases, a fatal complication.

The preventive aspect of malaria is as important as the curative one. Protection from mosquito bites is essential. Stagnant pools of water should be eliminated or sprayed over with an oil, the film of which precludes the multiplication of the malarial parasites. Spraying of chemical substances is, of course, important, but recent experience has shown that the parasite has developed resistance to insecticides used to kill it. Keeping the body covered at all hours of the day or night against mosquito bites is, therefore, more important.

Home Remedies: Cold water should be taken in adequate quantities, and if the temperature persists above 40°C, cold compresses should be applied to the forehead. In case of very high temperature—about 41.7°C or above—the patient should be wrapped in a sheet dipped in ice-cold water. The sheet should be removed after the coolness has been absorbed, dipped in water again, and rewrapped around the patient again. This process should be discontinued after the fever has come down to 39°C.

If the juice of 12 gm of holy basil (*tulsi*) is mixed with 3 gm black pepper powder and given to the patient during the cold stage of the fever, it will reduce the virulence of the hot stage when it occurs. Remember that holy basil is a good prophylactic agent against malaria and has been used in India for centuries now. Some Ayurvedic practitioners recommend the infusion of some leaves of *tulsi* and a couple of black peppers with one's tea as they can help stave off malaria. Even if the disease attacks, its severity would be reduced in a person who has been taking this infusion.

61

Medicines and Prescriptions:

1. *Sheetmani Rasa.* — 240 mg to be taken thrice daily with honey.

2. *Mahajwaarankusha Rasa, Shuddha Sphatika (alum).* — 120 mg of *Mahajwaarankusha Rasa* and 240 mg of *Shuddha Sphatika* to be taken thrice daily with juice of *tulsi* leaves.

The above medicines are for the first attacks of malaria; when the attacks are intermittent, the following medicines would be more useful:

1. *Tuvrimallayoga.* — 60 mg to be administered twice daily; the first dose should be given one hour before the attack and the other, one hour after.

2. *Godanti Bhasma; Shuddha Sphatika; Flesh of Karanja.* — 120 mg each of *Godanti Bhasma, Shuddha Sphatika* and flesh of *Karanja* should be made into 6 pills and taken at two-hourly intervals before the expected attack.

In the case of remittent fever, that is, one which continues without let-up, the following medicines are recommended:

1. *Jwarankusha; Tala Bhasma; Karanja Churna.* — 120 mg of *Jwarankusha,* 240 mg of *Talam Bhasma,* and 500 mg of *Karanja Churna* to be taken thrice daily with juice of *tulsi* leaves.

2. *Vishmushtyadi Vati or Karanjadi Vati; Talam Bhasma.* — 240 mg each of *Karanjadi Vati* and *Talam Bhasma* to be taken thrice daily with juice of *tulsi* leaves.

3. *Sudarshana Churna;*   2 gm *Sudarshana Churna*,
   Sphatika;   240 mg *Sphatika*, and 500
   Sarjika (soda-bicarb) mg *Sarjika* to be taken
                                 twice daily with warm
                                 water.

Diet and Other Regimen: Solid foods should be replaced by a liquid diet. Green vegetables and fruits are recommended in the post-recovery stage.

If a mild laxative is administered to the patient before an attack comes on, its virulence is modified. Daily activities should be increased only gradually.

Black-Water Fever[1] *(Kalamcha Jwara)*

Black-water fever is a complication of malaria characterised by haemoglobinuria (black water), the presence of blood pigment in the urine.

Causes and Symptoms: Black-water fever destroys the red blood corpuscles, resulting in the urine turning a dark red colour. It is an acute disease and generally occurs in tropical countries. Central Africa, India, and the Far East are susceptible areas. Ayurveda maintains that black-water fever is a result of the vitiation of *vata* and *kapha.*

The cardinal symptoms of black water fever are: temperature of the body ranging from 40° to 40.6°C, rigor or shivering, nausea, bilious vomiting, gastric discomfort, jaundice, and the passage of blackish or brownish urine due to the presence of the blood pigment in the urine. Both the spleen and the liver are enlarged and tender. The temperature of black-water fever falls after a few hours. It is preceded by profuse sweating, and the skin becomes jaundiced. Mild cases may recover in a couple of days but if there is delayed diagnosis or carelessness in the initiation of the treatment, the fever may last for many days. There may be a succession of attacks emaciating the patient. The disease occurs mostly in cases where quinine has been administered for a long period.

---

1. Readers are cautioned not to confuse black-water fever with kala-azar which is a totally different fever.

63

Home Remedies: The patient should be kept warm. A mild laxative or a soap water enema may be given to deal with constipation which is generally present. Water from a fresh coconut should be drunk instead of water.

Medicines & Prescriptions: The following medicines are recommended at the time the fever is at its height:

1. *Raktapittakulakandana Rasa; Chandanadi Lauha; Karanjadi Vati; Laksha Churna.* — 120 mg *Raktapittakulakananda*, 240 mg *Chandanadi Lauha,* and 500 mg each of *Karanjadi Vati* and *Laksha Churna* should be taken four times daily with decoction of bark of *neem.*

2. *Meghnada Rasa; Swarnamakshika Bhasma; Talbhasma; Swarnagairika.* — 120 mg each of *Meghnada Rasa, Swarnamakshika Bhasma,* and *Talbhasma*; along with 240 mg *Swarnagairika* should be taken four times a day.

Diet and Other Regimen: Sweet substances and liquids like sugarcane juice, fruit juice, and dry grapes should form the mainstay of the patient's diet. Spices, fats, tobacco, and alcohol are contraindicated.

Strict bedrest is advised for the patient.

Kala-Azar *(Kala Jwara)*

Kala-azar is also known as visceral leishmaniasis, Dum Dum Fever, and Black fever. The Assamese population of India calls it 'black disease'. It is a chronic disease which occurs along the shores of the Mediterranean, North Africa, Sudan, Assam in India, China, and the tropical zone of South America.

Causes and Symptoms: Allopaths believe that kala-azar is caused by an organism transmitted by the bite of a sandfly, usually the *Phlebotomus argentipes.*

The onset of kala-azar is acute or insidious, according to the virulence of the infection. There is irregular fever, progressive anaemia in which the white blood cells are found to be diminished, and marked enlargement of the spleen. The spleen of a kala-azar patient is sometimes found to weigh four to five kilograms.

The onset of fever in kala-azar, as has been mentioned above, is insidious. The fever rises gradually. But in about 25% of cases, the attack is sudden, the temperature reaching 104°C within a couple of hours. The fever attacks twice or three times in twenty-four hours. That is what distinguishes it from other intermittent fevers. It is irregular and may leave the patient after three to six weeks. But it recurs and leads to enlargement of the liver and the spleen, the former less than the latter. Many patients suffer from blue or black spots on their forehead, face, palms, or soles of the feet. A continuous distension of the stomach is also noticed. There is emaciation if the attacks continue, and there is a constant pain in the bones of the arms and the legs. The appetite of the patient is generally not affected and that probably explains the long course of the disease.

Medicines & Prescriptions:

1. *Shuddha Nilanjan (antimony); Mukta Bhasma; Praval Bhasma; Shuddha Swarnagairika; Shankha Bhasma.*

   60 mg each of *Shuddha Nilanjan* and *Mukta Bhasma;* and 120 mg each of *Praval Bhasma, Shuddha Swarnagairika,* and *Shankha Bhasma*— all to be taken four times daily with honey.

2. *Tamra Bhasma; Yakritaplihodaradilauha.*

   60 mg each of *Tamra Bhasma* and *Yakritaplihodaradilauha* to be taken twice daily, at midday and at night with honey.

Diet and Other Regimen: Nourishing food such as milk, milk products, eggs, fruits, and vegetables should be given to the patient in keeping with his condition.

Excessive physical exertion should be avoided.

Filariasis *(Shlipada Jwara)*

Filariasis occurs commonly in the Terai regions of the Himalayas, eastern Uttar Pradesh, Bihar, Bengal, Cochin, and Travancore,—all areas where natural drainage is defective, where water has a tendency to collect in pools and ponds, and where filaria-carrying mosquitoes are found in abundance.

Causes and Symptoms: According to allopathy, filariasis is caused by *Wuchereria bancrofti.* It is a threadlike worm. The female of the species is at least four feet long. The disease is transmitted to humans through contaminated water by infected mosquitoes. Once attacked, the person may not feel anything for almost a year, after which there is a painful swelling of the legs. The skin of the affected parts may become like that of an elephant—hence the name, elephantiasis. There is inflammation of the skin and the subcutaneous tissue, and concurrent obstruction of the lymphatic vessels. The thickening is due to excessive increase in the connective tissues. The inflammation also attacks the muscles of the legs and they become weak.

In some cases, there is involvement of the testicles which become inflamed and enlarged. Gross enlargement of the legs may take place to such an extent that their circumference increases to several times the normal size, and the scrotum may attain a weight of even upto twenty-five kilograms. Elephantiasis may develop elsewhere in the body, as in the arms, but the legs are the most commonly-affected parts.

Filariasis fever is a short, sharp fever. It rarely continues for more than four days, but its attacks are frequent. The inflammation tends to increase the size of the legs with each fresh attack. The testicles enlarge to enormous proportions and the patient has difficulty in walking, both on account of the increased circumference of the legs and the weakness of the muscles.

According to Ayurveda, the disease is caused by the vitiation of all the three *doshas*, but mainly *kapha*. Blood-letting is advised by the *acharya* in certain cases of elephantiasis, but it has to be done under the guidance of an expert.

Medicines & Prescriptions: For the fever which accompanies filariasis or elephantiasis, the following medicines are recommended:

Sanjivani;	120 mg each of *Sanjivani,*
Shringa Bhasma;	*Shringa Bhasma,* and
Hinguleshwar.	*Hinguleshwar* to be taken thrice daily with warm water.

After the fever has subsided, the following medicines should be tried for a permanent cure:

1. *Nityananda Rasa; Pippali Churna.*	250 mg of *Nityananda Rasa* and 500 mg of *Pippali Churna* to be taken twice (morning and midday) with decoction of bark of *Shakhotaka* tree.
2. *Shripadagajakeshari.*	120 mg should be given in one dose at night.

Home Remedies: A paste made of *Dhatur,* a root of the castor tree, *nirgundi, punarnava,* bark of *Sahijan* or mustard seeds—all in equal quantities—ground in cow urine or water should be applied over the affected parts.

Diet and Other Regimen: No diet restrictions are necessary. However hard-to-digest foods should be avoided.

The patient should ensure that he does not get any mosquito bites so as to avoid subsequent attacks.

Diseases of the Respiratory Organs

कामं प्राणहरा रोगा बहवो न तु ते तथा ।
यथा श्वासश्च हिक्का च प्राणानाशु निकृन्तत: ।।

*Although there are many diseases which destroy human life,
there are none that terminate it faster than hiccup and dyspnoea.*

CHARAKA SAMHITA

RESPIRATION IS the process in which air passes into and out of
the lungs with the object of allowing the blood to absorb oxygen
and give off carbon dioxide and water. The main parts of the
respiratory tract are: the nose, the throat, the larynx, the trachea
or the windpipe, the bronchi or bronchial tubes, and the lungs.

Diseases of the Nose

The nose is not only the upper part of the passage through
which air enters the lungs; it also lodges the organ which
furnishes the sense of smell. The outer part of the nose is not
of much importance except aesthetically; it is the inner organ—
the main part of the cavity which is placed above the roof of
the mouth—which is the real nose. The diseases to which the
nose is susceptible are many, the chief among them being
rhinitis (inflammation) which may become chronic if not treated
in time. According to Ayurveda, the number of diseases relating
to the nose is thirty-four. About a dozen of them are various
forms of inflammation and the rest pertain to tumours or
boils from which pus oozes out or foul-smelling phlegm is
produced.

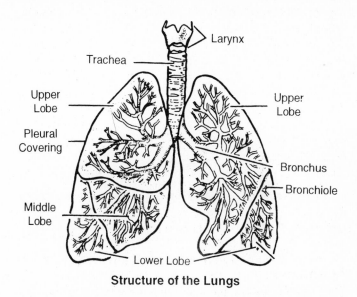

Structure of the Lungs

Common Cold *(Pratishyaya)*

The main villain of the piece behind diseases relating to the nose is the common cold. Coryza or catarrh of the nose is a common condition found in cold climates and during the change of season in countries like India. This is an irritating condition which is not fatal, but if neglected for a long time, it can create complications best avoided by timely attention. The common cold is generally treated lightly both by patients and physicians as is clear from the old adage: 'If you take medicine for a cold, it cures in a week, otherwise it takes seven days'.

Causes and Symptoms: Ayurveda has recognised five types of cold or *Pratishyaya* as those borne out of *vata*; borne out of the vitiation of *pitta*; borne out of *kapha*; borne out of disorders of the blood; and chronic cold borne out of the three *doshas*.

Home Remedies: In the case of a running nose, smoke from burning turmeric should be inhaled; it will encourage a copious discharge and shortly provide relief. Smoke from the root of *amaltas* also provides quick relief. *Jaiphala* (nutmeg) and cow's milk, sufficient to make a paste, together with 75 mg of opium should be applied to the forehead and the nose. In case the nose is blocked and the patient is unable to eject the phlegm, a powder of equal parts of cinnamon, black pepper, cardamom, and seeds of *krishnajiraka (Nigella sativa)* should be sniffed to induce sneezing. Decoction of bran should be taken at bedtime in a dose of 60 ml. Six grams of garlic and an equal quantity of gur pounded together may be given at bedtime.

Medicines & Prescriptions: *Laxmivilas Churna* and *Shring Bhasma* (calx of the horn) in quantities of 120 mg each, along with 240 mg *Narsar*, should be taken thrice daily with warm water.

Vyoshadi Vati should be sucked as a lozenge three to four times in the day.

In chronic coryza, the Ayurvedic medicines to be used are:

1. *Mahalaxmi Vilas.*	120 mg to be taken with powder of *mulethi*, honey, and *ghee*.
2. *Chitrak Hiratiki.*	10 gm to be taken in the morning and last thing at night with one cup of warm cow's milk.
3. *Vyoshadya Churna.*	3 gm to be taken twice with warm water after meals.
4. *Madhuyasthyadi Quath.*	50 ml to be taken thrice daily.

Diet & Other Regimen: A person suffering from a cold should be encouraged to take meat soup, vegetables with a bitter or sour taste, garlic, liquor in moderate quantities, and warm water. He should avoid heavily spiced or fried foods, and if the nostrils are dry and caked, he should take a large quantity of curds.

The patient should avoid a cold bath, particularly, of the head.

Nosebleed *(Nakseer)*

It is not uncommon for children or even adults to have an occasional nosebleed.

Causes and Symptoms: According to Ayurveda, bleeding from the nose is due to vitiation of *pitta*. If *pitta* has a tendency to go up, it may cause bleeding from the nose.

Home Remedies: Bleeding from the nose is not usually a very serious condition. In an ordinary nosebleed, the patient should be asked to lie still, and a cold compress should be applied to his head, which should be placed at a level lower than his feet. He should be asked to inhale iced water and refrain from blowing his nose. If this does not help, a few drops of the *swaras* (juice) of any of the following should be dropped into the nasal passage: onions, dub grass, tender flowers of the pomegranate tree, shelled mango seeds, or jwasa (*Alhagi pseudalbagi*).

In case bleeding is very severe and the patient appears to be losing too much of blood, gauze soaked with *panchkshiri kashaya* or alum (*phitkiri*), camphor, and *majuphala* in equal quantities and in powder form should be dropped into the nose. *Amla* should be ground in buttermilk and the paste should be put in a little boiling ghee. When it is cold, it should be applied to the forehead and the outside of the nose.

Surgical Remedies: Sushruta has advised that in case all the remedies described above fail to ameliorate the condition and bleeding continues, posing a danger to the life of a patient, recourse should be taken to surgery. It is possible that a blood vessel in the organ may have burst. Electric cauterization is the final remedy.

In case the nosebleed is due to high blood pressure, drugs to reduce it should be administered.

71

Influenza *(Vata Sleshmika Jwara)*

Influenza is an acute infectious disease of which there have been several epidemics. In the twentieth century itself, five massive epidemics have been recorded which have taken a heavy toll of human life. The severest epidemic was during 1918-19, when fifteen to twenty million people died throughout the world.

Causes and Symptoms: Allopaths believe that influenza is caused by a virus, and suggest an incubation period of one to ten days, depending on the severity of the attack. Influenza generally strikes at the change of seasons. Ayurveda believes that the balance of the three *doshas—vata, pitta,* and *kapha—* is disturbed when the seasons are changing. Persons who are prone to suffering from constipation, or from diseases of the mucus membrane of the nasal passage or the throat, are more susceptible to influenza.

The onset of influenza is sudden. It is characterized by fever ranging between 38.3°C to 39.4°C, headache, sore throat, coryza with sneezing, pains all over the body, and restlessness.

The cardinal symptoms of influenza are: irritation, and later, inflammation of the nose, pharynx, and larynx; nose bleed; and a dry hacking cough. In the later stages of the disease, there may be involvement of the lungs, particularly among elderly patients. The disease is marked by extreme prostration, and even after recovery, the sufferer has to undergo a long period of convalescence.

Home Remedies: Long pepper (*pippali*) is one of the best remedies for influenza and troubles associated with it. Half a teaspoonful of powder of long pepper, mixed with two teaspoonfuls of honey and half a teaspoonful of ginger juice— administered thrice during the day, will effectively counteract the onset of influenza. The preparation is particularly useful in avoiding complications which follow the onset of the disease, namely, the involvement of the larynx and the bronchial tubes. The other remedy recommended is the green leaves of the *tulsi* plant (*Ocimum sanctum*). About 1 gm of these leaves and dry ginger should be boiled, and the decoction taken as tea. Sugar may be added according to taste. Incidentally, the leaves of the plant are also helpful in preventing malaria and other seasonal fevers. A few leaves may be boiled with tea, and the decoction taken twice at teatime.

Yet another effective remedy for influenza is *haridra* (turmeric). A teaspoonful of the powder or paste of turmeric should be added to a cup of warm milk and taken with sugar, thrice during the day. It prevents lung complications and also activates the liver, which has a tendency to become sluggish during an attack of influenza. If the fever is accompanied by a cough, a teaspoonful of ginger juice should be added.

Medicines & Prescriptions: Two tablets of *Tribhuvana Kirtirasa*, of 75 mg each, should be taken with one teaspoon of honey, three to four times a day.

Diet and Other Regimen: The patient should not be given any solids for the first twenty-four hours of the onset of the disease. Sago boiled in water or milk may be given to sustain his strength. Soups of vegetables and meat can supplement his diet. Garlic fried in ghee or butter, or in a raw form, is also helpful. Heavy foods should be avoided. Fruits like banana, guava and those with a sour taste should be prohibited. If the patient is addicted to tea, he should be advised to replace it with coffee or asked to add *tulsi* leaves or *banafsha* flowers to the tea.

Exposure to cold, bathing, physical labour, and sleeplessness should be avoided as they tend to aggravate the condition. A mild laxative is also indicated in most cases.

Cough and Disorders of the Throat *(Kasa Roga)*

The throat, in popular language, is the term applied to the region in front of the neck. The correct description is the pharynx and the cavity at the back of the mouth, into which the nose, the mouth, the wind pipe, the food pipe, and the Eustachian tubes open.

In Ayurveda, however, the diseases of this region of the body are treated under the general head—*Kasa Roga.*

Causes and Symptoms: *Kasa Roga* is sub-divided into five heads: disorders borne out of *vata, pitta, kapha* or phlegm, injuries or infections, and those caused by tuberculosis. The first three types are easily handled, but the latter two categories are a different proposition altogether. But whatever the type of *kasa*, if it is allowed to persist, it becomes chronic and may even result in consumption or tuberculosis. Clinically, the diseases may be distinguishable from each other, but practically, *kasa roga* is broadly of three types: cough without expectoration; cough with expectoration; and cough mixed with blood, which occurs in typical cases of pulmonary tuberculosis. Injuries or infections in the region of the throat might also produce blood-mixed phlegm which is a serious condition.

Ayurveda has categorized what modern medicine calls bronchitis into another type of *kasa roga*; it may be acute or it may turn chronic and deteriorate into tubercular bronchitis. In some cases, particularly among the aged, the lack of elasticity in the lung tissues or lung fibrosis may turn into *bronchiectasis*.

Diseases of the throat may be of respiratory origin or of an extra-respiratory character. Pharyngitis, tonsillitis, and adenoids are disorders not directly connected with the process of respiration, even though we propose to treat them under this head.

Home Remedies: In coughs where there is no expectoration, that is, no phlegm is produced, the treatment should start with the lubrication of the throat. Ayurvedic practitioners advise such patients to consume milk and *ghee*. A decoction of liquorice root (*mulethi* or *madhuka*) should be given with sugar or honey to clear the phlegm. Another common remedy is black pepper in doses of 250 to 750 mg, given with *ghee*, sugar, and honey. A paste made of equal parts of black raisins, dates, black pepper, *vidanga* (*bahera*), long pepper (*pippali*), and honey should be used to get quick relief. Alternatively, a linctus made of the powder of long pepper, ginger, nut grass (*nagarmusta*), *harada*, and sugar or honey can be taken with advantage.

Medicines and Prescriptions: Standard Ayurvedic medicines used in cough are: *Chaturashana Churna, Eladi Churna,* and *Yavani Shadava.* The dosage and duration of treatment are indicated on the packing of the drug; they also depend on the severity of the disease and response to treatment.

Diet and Other Regimen: The dietary regimen to be followed in cases of cough and allied disorders is to encourage the use of wheat, *moong* (green gram), old rice, barley, goat's milk, cow's milk, *ghee*, soup of mutton or venison, raisins, and *amla.* One should avoid *bael* fruit, brinjal, bitter gourd, mustard, fried artichoke.

The patient should desist from sexual intercourse and avoid sleep during the day. If there is constipation, a laxative such as castor oil should be taken.

Whooping Cough *(Dushta Kasa)*

Whooping cough is known as *dushta kasa* in Ayurveda. It is an infectious bacterial disease, which occurs mainly in children.

Causes and Symptoms: Allopaths believe whooping cough to be a result of infection caused by the organism *Bordetella pertussis.* In the beginning, it is marked by catarrh of the nose, sneezing, watering of the eyes, irritation of the throat, feverishness, and cough. Later, the symptoms of catarrh disappear but the cough becomes more persistent. The cough is marked by paroxysms of coughing, consisting of a series of violent and rapid expiratory coughs, succeeded by a loud, sonorous or crowing inspiration—the whoop—hence the name, whooping cough. The patient sometimes turns blue in the face because the paroxysm deprives his lungs of air. Children are usually more susceptible to the malady than adults. According to Ayurveda, whooping cough is the result of disturbance of the *vata dosha* in the body.

Medicines & Prescriptions: The best remedies for whooping cough are *Aparajita Leha*, *Dashamuli Ghrita*, *Kantakaryavaleh,* and *Panchmuli Kashaya.*

These may be taken as indicated on the packing or as prescribed by the physician.

Home Remedies: Juice of ginger (14 ml), with an equal quantity of honey, taken twice a day is also helpful.

Diet and Other Regimen: The dietary regimen for whooping cough is the same as prescribed for dry, hacking coughs or disorders of the throat.

Castor oil should be administered occasionally to the patient to relieve his constipation, and also to relieve the pain he is liable to feel because the paroxysms make his abdominal muscles tender. The patient must be protected against exposure and sudden colds as they are liable to aggravate his condition and hamper a quick recovery.

Bronchitis *(Shwasa Pranali Shoth)*

A serious variety of *kasa roga*, bronchitis is characterised by inflammation of the bronchial tubes which carry air to the lungs. This disease is endemic to cold damp climates but may strike anywhere.

Causes and Symptoms: Even though it is caused by certain germs, the susceptibility of certain constitutions cannot be denied. Ayurveda ascribes it to impairment of the digestive processes, and the remedies selected for its cure are those which help restore the digestive balance too.

There is inflammation of the mucous membrane of the bronchi to which phlegm adheres, and there is difficulty in expelling it. The phlegm, when expelled, is found to be viscid and may be purulent. Due to the tendency of the viscid phlegm to stick to the bronchi, there is difficulty in breathing and the lungs are starved of air. A fit of coughing may turn the face of the patient blue. Bronchitis patients are thin and emaciated. In its acute form, bronchitis may result in a rise of temperature, breathlessness, and loss of appetite. If proper care is not taken and the disease becomes chronic, it may deteriorate into continuous breathlessness.

Home Remedies: The simplest treatment for bronchitis is administration of one teaspoonful of turmeric powder (*haridra*) with a glass of milk, twice or thrice daily. It acts best when taken on an empty stomach. A powder of equal quantities of dried ginger, black pepper, and long pepper (*pippali*) can be given thrice daily. It may be mixed with honey or infused with your daily tea. Its anti-pyretic qualities deal with the fever attendant upon bronchitis and also tone up the metabolism of the patient. Juice of *vasa* (*Adhatoda vasica*) may be taken thrice daily, in two teaspoonful doses. Two teaspoonfuls of honey taken daily are also helpful in bronchitis.

Medicines & Prescriptions: Some well-known Ayurvedic preparations for bronchitis, both acute and chronic, are given below:

1. *Rasa Sindur;* *Pravala Pisthi;* *Sitopaladi Churna.*	120 mg *Rasa Sindur*, 240 mg *Pravala Pisthi*, and 3 gm *Sitopaladi Churna* to be taken thrice daily with *ghee*.
2. *Kaphachintamani;* *Kaphaketu;* *Shringyadi Churna.*	120 mg each of *Kapha-chintamani* and *Kaphaketu*, and 2 gm of *Shringyadi Churna* to be taken thrice daily.

In case of a congested throat which accompanies bronchitis in many cases, *Khadiradi Vati* should be sucked as a lozenge five times a day. The main ingredient of the drug, catechu, helps relieve the congestion.

Diet and Other Regimen: Curds and sour substances should be avoided. Banana and guava are fruits which are contraindicated in this malady.

Smoking is contraindicated and consumption of liquor should be reduced to the minimum, Excessive physical exercise and exposure to cold and damp should be avoided.

Bronchial Asthma (*Tomaka Shvasa*)

Bronchial asthma is known as *Tomaka Shvasa* in Ayurveda. It is on the rise today, with increasing levels of pollution and the stressful lifestyle followed by people.

Causes and Symptoms: Bronchial asthma is supposed to originate from afflictions of the stomach and the gastro-intestinal tract. That is why in the preliminary stage of the disease or just before its onset, the patient complains of indigestion, constipation, or diarrhoea. The attack of asthma may come without warning because of the hypersensitivity of the patient to certain substances like pollen, dust, emanations from certain animals like dogs and cats, certain foods to which the person is allergic and, of course, certain bacteria.

Asthma is characterised by difficulty in breathing, a sense of tightness, constriction around the chest, and a wheezing noise as the breath is expelled. The small bronchial tubes which connect with the lungs are constricted due to swelling or accumulation of viscid phlegm in the main bronchi, hence the difficulty in inspiration and expiration.

The attack of asthma comes on in the early morning when the patient suddenly wakes up with a feeling of apprehension and alarm. He sits up as the breathing suddenly becomes impossible in a recumbent position. He may rush to open the window as it becomes difficult to breathe in a closed room. The attack may last for a few hours or a few days before it subsides, and, in the early stages of the disease, the patient feels normal after the attack. It is only when it becomes chronic that he acquires a typical asthmatic look--a pale face and an emaciated body.

Medicines & Prescriptions: Well-known preparations for this disease in Ayurveda are *Chyavanaprash* and *Agastya Rasayana*. The main ingredient of the former medicine is *amla,* the richest source of Vitamin C in nature. A peculiarity of this fruit is that its vitamin content is not lost by exposure to heat as is the case with other drugs and fruits. The latter preparation is indicated in cases of asthma where the patient is constipated; in particularly emaciated sufferers, however, *Chyavanaprash* is the better remedy. Both the drugs can be taken in one teaspoonful doses thrice a day, preferably before food is ingested. They are slow-acting remedies but are surer in their efficacy. In chronic cases, their effect is evident from the increasing gap between successive attacks.

Along with the preparations mentioned above, *Sitopaladi Churna* should be taken thrice or four times a day in one teaspoonful doses with honey. Since the drug is likely to cause irritation of the throat, it is better when mixed with honey and taken as a linctus. Medicines containing minerals which are recommended in cases of asthma are: *Swasha-Kasa-Chintamani Rasa*, *Suvarna-Pushpasuga Rasa*, and *Kanakasava*. The dosage and duration of these medicines will depend upon the severity of the disease.

Any of the following prescriptions can be tried with the advice of the physician:

1. *Vasa Churna;* *Shukti Bhasma;* *Trikuti Churna.*	2 gm of *Vasa Churna*, 125 mg of *Shukti Bhasma*, and 1 gm *Trikuti Churna* should be taken thrice daily with honey.
2. *Old Gur;* *Mustard Oil.*	10 gm each of old *Gur* and *Mustard oil* to be taken daily.
3. *Bharangi;* *Nagara.*	2 gm each of *Bharangi* and *Nagara* should be ground into a paste with water and taken twice daily with warm water.

Diet and Other Regimen: The patient is advised to avoid curd, buttermilk, bananas, guavas, and fried foods. Light food should be taken at night and all sour substances should be banned.

Smoking is contraindicated and consumption of liquor should be reduced to the minimum. Excessive physical exercise and exposure to cold and damp should be avoided.

Tonsillitis *(Tundikeri)*

Tonsillitis is the inflammation of the tonsils—the small rounded masses of mainly lymphoid tissues behind the tongue, on either side of the pharynx.

Causes and Symptoms: Latest research has reached the conclusion that the tonsils act as barriers to infection. The mechanism whereby they tend to fight infection has not yet been identified, but observations have confirmed the view that children whose tonsils have been removed are more susceptible to infections than others. A body of opinion has therefore arisen which frowns upon surgical interference in obstinate cases of tonsillitis.

The onset of tonsillitis is manifested by a pain in swallowing, a sensation of chill, and fever. On visual examination, the tonsils are found to be enlarged, engorged, and covered with a varying amount of whitish or grey material—the purulent discharge. Inflammation is not restricted to the tonsils and, generally, the entire throat is involved. The glands under the jaws are also inflamed and tender to the touch. In severe cases there may be pain in the ear. These symptoms, particularly in children and adolescents upto the age of eighteen years, might be the precursor of rheumatic fever, a serious condition.

Since it is usually associated with attacks of cough and cold, Ayurvedists call the disease *Tundikeri* or *Galayu*. Constipation and other disorders of the digestive system are liable to precipitate the attack. In severe cases, there may be difficulty in breathing in addition to fever and a coated tongue.

Home Remedies: The treatment of tonsillitis must start with hot fomentation of the front of the neck and steps should be taken to keep the region warm. Twelve grams of *banafsha* flowers (*Viola odorata*) boiled in 50 ml of milk is a useful home remedy for tonsillitis. The milk should be filtered and drunk. The filtered *banafsha* should be lightly fried in *ghee* and worn round the throat as a poultice at night. Decoction of the bark of the acacia (*babul*) tree mixed with rock salt should be used for gargles. If that is not easy to come by, saline gargles should be resorted to. The powder of *Vasti Madhu* (*Glycyrrhiza glabra*), *Vacha* (*Acorus calamus*), and *Kulanjana* (*Alipina galanga*), made into a paste with honey, should be used as a linctus. Roots of *Vacha* (*Acorus calamus*) and *Sati* (*Curcuma zedoria*) may be ground in milk and a paste prepared. It can be used as nasal drops to relieve the congestion of the nose.

Medicines & Prescriptions:

1. *Khadiradi Vati.*	Six tablets to be sucked daily as lozenges.
2. *Agastya Rasayana.*	Take twice daily with honey in dosage as prescribed by the doctor.

A continued use of *Agastya Rasayana* for about six months will grant immunity from the disease for life.

Diet and Other Regimen: Soup of meat and lentils like *moong* are recommended for patients suffering from tonsillitis. Bland soft foods, gruel, and lukewarm liquids are the best. Chillies and other condiments should be avoided as they tend to irritate the throat. Vegetables like bitter gourd, fenugreek (*methi*), and young radishes are particularly recommended. Sour substances, curds, buttermilk, and fried foods are to be avoided.

Warm saline gargles are recommended twice a day.

Hoarseness *(Swarabheda)*

Hoarseness of the voice is a complaint which accompanies or results from laryngitis (the inflammation of the larynx).

Causes and Symptoms: Hoarseness may be caused by certain infections, taking of hot and cold substances alternately, or any abnormal growth and infection produced by chronic tuberculosis. In addition to difficulty in articulation, the patient suffers from a coated tongue, pain on swallowing, and, sometimes, fever accompanied by a burning sensation in the throat. Constipation tends to aggravate the condition.

Home Remedies: Powder of *Vasti Madhu* and *Vacha* should be given in one teaspoonful doses thrice a day with honey. Saline gargles or gargles with the decoction of the bark of the acacia tree are recommended as a palliative.

Medicines & Prescriptions: *Khadiradi Vati* or *Eladi Vati* should be sucked as lozenges.

Diet and Other Regimen: Chillies and other condiments should be avoided, as also sour, heavy, fatty foods.

Any strain on the voice should be avoided as far as possible.

Tuberculosis (*Rajayakshma*)

Tuberculosis is the king of diseases. According to Hindu mythology, the Moon, the king among the satellites of the earth, was afflicted by a curse of Brahma, the creator, and hence the name, *Rajayakshma*.

Tuberculosis is one of the most highly contagious diseases to have afflicted mankind.

Causes and Symptoms: Tuberculosis, or TB in popular parlance, is caused by the tiny organism, *Mycobacterium tuberculosis*. Little lumps or tubercles form in the part affected, and become soft and suppurate as the disease advances. A slight rise in temperature—generally in the evening, night sweats, discharge of blood with phlegm, and extensive bleeding from the lungs in the final stages, bring on death. TB may affect the bones, the membranes of the brain (leading to meningitis), or the glands, when it is called scrofula. It may be caused when a person pricks himself with anything sharp infected with the germs, or inhalation of dust particles mixed with the tiny microbe. But the main factor responsible for the disease is the susceptibility to it, due to a constitution weakened by continuous ill health, a lowered power of resistance, heredity, an unhealthy atmosphere, excessive use of intoxicants, over-indulgence in sex, asthma, and a disease of the metabolism like diabetes. It is also a disease connected with filth and poverty and does not usually attack persons living in clean surroundings and having sufficient means to feed themselves properly.

In the early stages of the disease, there is an irritating cough, particularly in the morning, either without an expectoration or with a clear mucus or phlegm. The first sign of the disease is blood-flecked phlegm attended by fever in the evenings and below normal temperature in the early morning. There are also night sweats. When the symptoms are aggravated and emaciation has set in, the second stage is supposed to have been reached. If extreme care is not taken and treatment is not initiated, it may spread to the throat and the intestines. The terminal stage comes when the illness reaches deep into the lungs and they are full of cavities. The voice of the patient may become husky at this stage; there may be diahorrea and extreme prostration, with the patient being unable to leave the bed. Death comes because of extensive haemorrhage.

The duration of the illness depends on four factors: the intensity of the infection; the age of the patient; the stage at which the disease has been recognised; and the natural resistance of the body.

Types of Tuberculosis: If the disease reaches the intestines, there is inflammation of the bowels with impairment of digestion, loss of appetite, distension of the stomach, rumbling noises in the abdomen and a persistent ache. If the small intestine is involved, the patient is constipated, but when the large intestine is the seat of the malady, diahorrea is the result. Emaciation increases faster than in pulmonary TB.

In scrofula or TB of the glands, inflammation is the chief characteristic. The glands are swollen and enlarged and they suppurate.

When a patient suffers from TB of the bones, the bones start crumbling. If the disease reaches the spine, there is curvature and the patient is unable to stand erect. TB of the bones generally affects young people. In older people, the bones generally affected are the femur and the tibia.

Tuberculosis of the Lungs

Pulmonary tuberculosis or phthisis is the most dangerous type of tuberculosis. Little lumps or tubercles form in the lungs. The affected part becomes soft and suppurates as the disease advances. A slight rise of temperature—generally in the evenings, night sweats, discharge of blood with phlegm, and extensive bleeding from the lungs in the final stages, bring on death.

The preventive aspect of tuberculosis is more social than medical. It is from the slums that the disease starts its fatal march. Provision of clean, healthy surroundings with properly ventilated and clean houses is the first imperative. Detection and isolation of the victims of the disease is the second most important thing that should be done. Thirdly, the diet is of primary importance. Plenty of milk, butter, eggs, black gram or its pulse, gourds of the various varieties, turnips, beetroot, spinach and other green vegetables, and fruits are the other preventives. As has been stated earlier, tuberculosis is a disease of filth and poverty. Clean surroundings are a must if TB is to be prevented.

Home Remedies: The treatment of a case of pulmonary tuberculosis must start with the isolation of the patient and his removal to a sanitorium if the disease has been detected at a secondary stage. If that is not possible, he should be housed in an airy room where there is plenty of sunlight. Sunlight is important because the germs causing the disease fall victim only to direct sunlight; neither boiling nor freezing makes them ineffective.

Ayurveda recommends *Vasa* (*Adhotoda vasica*) for tuberculosis. One ounce of the juice from the leaves of the drug given thrice a day with honey provides relief. *Rudanti* (*Cressa crestca*) given in 2 gm doses twice daily, reduces the severity of the disease. Garlic is another wonderful drug in the cure of TB. Thirty grains of garlic boiled in about eight ounces of milk and two pounds of water should be administered in two doses during the day. But the medicine is ready only when the whole decoction has been reduced to one fourth of its original quantity.

Medicines & Prescriptions: The preparation of choice is *Naradiya Mahalakshami Vilasa Rasa* which contains traces of gold. It should be administered in three doses of 200 mg each in the day. *Swarna Vasanta Malati* is the preparation used in cases where there is excessive fever, sweating, and a burning sensation on the palms of the hands and the soles of the feet.

Drakshasava should be administered in one ounce doses after meals. It should be mixed with an equal quantity of water. *Chyavanaprash Avaleha* is another wonderful remedy that provides strength and sustenance to the patient. It also increases the appetite. The dosage in the beginning should be two teaspoonfuls with milk on an empty stomach twice daily, but as the patient gains strength, it should be increased.

When there is a dry cough accompanied by fever during the night, and weakness, the following prescription is recommended: *Suvarna Vasanta Malati Rasa*—250 mg, 500 mg of *Praval Pishti*, and 250 mg of *Amritasatva* should be taken with preserve of *amla* thrice daily.

In case of high temperature, either of the following prescriptions is recommended:

1. *Muktapanchamrita;* *Pachanana Rasa;* *Amritasatva.*	120 mg each of *Muktapanchamrita* and *Panchanana Rasa,* and 240 mg of *Amritasatva* to be taken morning and evening with honey.
2. *Chandramrita;* *Sitopaladi.*	1 gm *Chandramrita* and 12 gm *Sitopaladi* to be mixed with honey and used as a linctus.

In case there is blood-filled phlegm, the following prescriptions are recommended:

1. *Vasantamalati;* *Raktapitta Kula-* *kandana Rasa;* *Shatamulyadi Loha;* *Lakshadi Churna;* *Sitopaladi.*	120 mg each of *Vasantamalati* and *Raktapitta Kulakandana Rasa,* 240 mg of *Shatamulyadi Loha,* and 1 gm each of *Lakshadi Churna* and *Sitopaladi* to be taken thrice daily with honey.
2. *Swarnamakshik* *Bhasma;* *Praval Pishti;* *Vasavaleha.*	120 mg *Swarnamakshik Bhasma,* 240 mg *Praval Pishti,* and 10 gm *Vasavakha* to be taken morning and evening with goat's milk.

Diet and Other Regimen: Dried fruits, particularly dried grapes and almond oil, are useful in this condition. Drumsticks, *patola,* and *kundru* are the best vegetables recommended for a consumptive patient. Goat's milk, flesh, and even urine, are useful for a TB patient. Substances which aggravate *kapha* like curds, buttermilk, bananas, and guavas should be banned.

No hard physical or mental exercise should be permitted. Living in airy surroundings and going for walks in the morning and evening are recommended. Sexual intercourse should be avoided as it is likely to aggravate the condition.

Hiccough *(Hikka Roga)*

Hiccough (Hiccups) is a spasmodic indrawing of air into the lungs, resulting in a whoop.

Causes and Symptoms: The cause, generally, is some irritation of the nerves of the diaphragm, which produces sudden contractions of the latter. Most cases are due to disorders of digestion, but the symptoms also occur in some serious diseases like the uraemia of Bright's disease. In such cases, it is a grave sign.

According to Ayurveda, the aggravation and upward movement of *vayu* is the primary cause of hiccups. A dietary irregularity or indiscretion, as also psychic factors like anxiety, nervousness, and anger may also cause hiccups, depending upon the *doshas* involved.

Home Remedies: The ash of the peacock feather is a specific remedy for this condition; 150 to 400 mg should be administered with honey six times during the day, depending upon the severity of the disease. Fomentation with a hot water bag is also recommended. Smoke from burning black gram and a piece of old rope should be inhaled at the beginning of an attack. A few mouthfuls of water swallowed suddenly may also relieve the condition.

Medicines & Prescriptions:

1. *Eladi Vati.*	Should be sucked six times daily or ground and mixed with honey and used as a linctus.
2. *Hingutriguna Taila.*	Should be used for massaging the abdomen.
3. *Sukumara Ghrita.*	One teaspoonful thrice daily with milk.

86

Psychotherapy is recommended if the condition is the result of psychological reasons.

Diet and Other Regimen: Fatty and heavy foods are to be avoided; a light, liquid diet is recommended.

If there is constipation present, it should be relieved by administration of laxatives.

Pneumonia *(Shwasanat Jwara)*

Pneumonia is the inflammation of one lung, whereas double pneumonia is inflammation of both the lungs. The air sacs are filled with thick secretions and become solid in the late stage of the disease.

Causes and Symptoms: As in most diseases, allopathy believes that pneumonia is caused by an organism, *pneumococcus,* which has an incubation period of two to six days. The attack usually begins with a fit of shivering, or, in the case of children, with convulsions. The temperature rises at once from 38.3°C to 39.4°C; the pulse is rapid, and breathing shallow and painful. There is coughing and the phlegm produced is sticky and, sometimes, flecked with blood. The temperature continues at about 40°C for about a week. After that, it has a tendency to fall suddenly, and the patient experiences copious perspiration and a sinking feeling with extreme prostration. Pain which accompanies the onset of the disease may cease, but sometimes travels to the pit of the stomach. This may confuse the physician, who may diagnose it to be of abdominal origin.

A pneumonia patient generally complains of sleeplessness, and the affected side of the chest may stop moving during inspiration and expiration. The whole situation is compounded if both the lungs are affected and double pneumonia develops. The disease sometimes leads to pleurisy or inflammation of the pleura, and collection of fluid in the pleural cavity, which is a serious condition.

Ayurveda believes that pneumonia is caused by the disturbance of the *vata dosha* in the body. The most critical period in the course of the disease is the crisis that may occur on the tenth day from the onset of the fever when the temperature suddenly falls to normal. The patient perspires profusely and there is extreme weakness with feeble breathing.

Medicines & Prescription: The following medicines are recommended during the initial stage of the disease:

1. *Shringa Bhasma; Rasa Sindur; Shringrabhra; Narsar.*	120 mg each of *Shringa Bhasma, Rasa Sindur,* and *Shringrabhra;* and 240 mg *Narsar* to be taken thrice daily with juice of ginger.
2. *Ashtadashang Quath.*	150 ml to be taken once daily in the morning.

If the patient has rapid breathing, the following medicines should be tried:

1. *Swash Kasa Chintamani; Mayura Pichha Bhasma; Rock Salt; Pippali Churna; Apamargakshara; Kakarasingi Churna.*	120 mg each of *Swash Kasa Chintamani, Mayura Pichha Bhasma, Rock Salt,* and *Pippali Churna;* 360 mg *Apamargakshara,* 5 gm *Kakarasingi Churna* should be taken four times a day with honey.
2. *Chandramrita; Yavakshara; Talishadi Churna.*	0.5 gm *Chandramrita,* 1 gm *Yavakshara,* and 6 gm *Talishadi Churna* should be mixed with 12 gm of syrup of *Lisora* (*Cordia mysa*) and used as a linctus.

In case there is accompanying delirium, preparations like *Vata Chintamani, Chaturbhuja Rasa, Shringabhasma, Tribhuvanakirti Rasa, Kasturibhairava Rasa, Naradeeya Laxmivilasa Rasa* should be given. *Dashanga Lepa* should be used for massaging the chest. The advice of the treating physician must be taken.

At the time of crisis (when the fever suddenly goes down), the following is the best prescription: *Visheshwar Rasa* and

Kasturibhairava in quantities of 120 mg each, and 180 mg of *Saubhagya Vati* should be taken six times with cardamom powder and honey.

Diet and Other Regimen: Diet should consist of light and easily-digestible foods. Warm soups are recommended.

Till the fever persists, the patient should keep himself protected against the cold. After the fever comes down, light exercise, starting with walking, is recommended.

विरोधीन्यन्नपानानि द्रवस्निग्धगुरूणि च ।
भजतामागतां छर्दिं वेगांश्चान्यान्प्रतिघ्नताम् ॥
व्यायाममतिसंतापमतिभुक्त्वोपसेविनाम् ।
शीतोष्णलंध.नाहारान् क्रमं मुक्त्वा निषेविणाम् ॥
घर्मश्रमभयार्तानां द्रुतं शीताम्बुसेविनाम् ।
अजीर्णाध्यशिनां चैव पञ्चकर्मापचारिणाम् ।
नवान्नदधिमत्स्यातिलवणाम्ल निषेविणाम् ।
माषमूलकपिष्टान्नति लक्षीरगुडाशिनाम् ॥
व्यवायं चाप्यजीर्णेऽन्ने निद्रां च भजतां दिवा ।
विप्रान् गुरून् धर्मयतां पापं कर्म च कुर्त्तताम् ॥
वातादयस्त्रयो दुष्टारत्वग्रक्तं मांसमम्बु च ।
दूषयन्ति स कुष्ठानां सप्तको द्रव्यसंग्रहः ॥

The constant use of mutually incompatible eats and drinks or liquid; unctuous and heavy articles of diet; the suppression of the generated urge for vomiting and other calls of nature; indulgence in exercise or exposure to heat after a surfeit meal; irregular indulgence in cold or hot food, or fasting or over-eating; using of cold water suddenly after being afflicted with heat, fatigue or fear; indulgence in pre-digestion meals; wrongful administration of the five purificatory procedures; habitual use of new grain, curds or fish; excessive use of salt, or acid articles, or of black gram, radish, pasted articles, til, milk, or gur, performing the sex-act before the ingested food is digested; day sleep; the persecution of wise men and elders; and the committing of sinful acts: by these factors, all the three humors—vata, pitta, *and* kapha, *which have become morbid, vitiate the skin, blood, flesh, and the body fluid. This is the complex of the seven body elements affected in dermatosis.*

CHARAKA SAMHITA

Diseases of the Skin & Hair

THE SKIN consists of two layers which differ in structure and in origin: the cuticle, also known as scarf-skin, epidermis, or epithelium; and the true skin, also known as *cutis vera*, corium, or dermis. The cuticle varies from a thickness of 0.1 mm to 1 mm. The true skin is the fibrous layer which forms the chief part of the body covering. It varies in thickness from 0.5 mm to 3 mm, being coarser on the back than in the front of the body, and thicker in men than in women. The skin contains two types of glands: sebaceous glands, which secrete a fatty substance; and sweat glands which secrete a clear, watery liquid. The main function of the skin is a protective one: it covers the underlying muscles, by both protecting them from injury, specially by virtue of the layer of fat immediately beneath the skin, and warding off extremes of temperature. The cuticle forms a highly impenetrable surface, its horny character and elasticity being well calculated to resist wounds, while the sebaceous matter with which it is provided, renders it almost water-proof. Thus, poisons and drugs are not absorbed in any appreciable amount through the unbroken skin, unless combined with some fatty material, as in ointments. The other functions of the skin are secretion, heat regulation, and respiration (particularly in lower animals).

Skin disorders fall into four categories: disorders of the secreting apparatus, disorders relating to growths on the skin, inflammatory infections, and nervous and parasitic infections. We shall deal with them in the order of their seriousness.

Leprosy *(Kushta Roga)*

Leprosy is a chronic disease which particularly affects the mucous membranes of the skin and nerves. The disease is mainly prevalent in Africa, the Indian sub-continent, the Far East, and Central and South America.

Causes and Symptoms: According to modern medicine the causative organism of leprosy is *Mycobacterium leprae*, discovered in 1872. There are two distinct types of leprosy: tuberculoid and lepromatous. The differentiation is important since the former runs a relatively benign course and is often self-healing, whereas the latter is a steadily progressive form of the disease. The distinction cannot, however, be always made because mixed symptoms are usually found. The symptoms involve the skin as well as the nervous system. The skin manifestations range from areas of whitening of the skin to massive nodules, such as are so often visible on the bodies of lepers. The nerve involvement may be that of pain in certain centres or, in serious cases, total loss of feeling in certain parts of the body. The eyes may be affected, leading to total blindness, and ulcers may occur in the mouth and the larynx. There are tragic cases of deformity when the fingers fall off at the joints, leaving only the palms over which the entire skin starts rotting.

Aggravation of all the three *doshas* of the body, according to Ayurveda, is the causative factor in leprosy. The two main divisions of *kushta roga* are: *mahakushta* which is of seven types, and *kshudra kushta* which is of eleven types. In the latter category are included leprous afflictions which are confined to the skin.

Eczema, ecthyosis—where the skin resembles the scales of a fish; xerodermia pigmentosa—where the skin is dry and resembles the skin of an elephant; psoriasis—in which the skin turns black and coarse; rhagades—splitting of the skin on the hands and feet; lichen—acute itch and boils; ringworm; excoriation—destruction of small areas of the surface of the skin or mucous membrane; scabies; bullae; erythemas—these are all the various forms of leprosy according to Ayurveda.

Medicines & Prescriptions:

1. *Rasamanikya; Gandhaka Rasayana; Panchanimba Churna.*	120 mg of *Rasamanikya*, 500 mg of *Gandhaka Rasayana*, and 1 gm of *Panchanimba Churna* to be taken in the morning and evening.
2. *Mahatiktaka Ghrita; Navakakashaya.*	12 ml *Mahatiktaka Ghrita* and 58 ml *Navakakashaya* to be taken twice daily after No. 1.
3. *Khadradirishta.*	24 ml to be taken twice daily, after meals, with lukewarm water.

Diet and Other Regimen: Only easy-to-digest foods should be taken.

Injuries to any part of the body, particularly, the hands and feet, should be avoided.

Eczema *(Vicharchika)*

Eczema, in Ayurveda, is a superficial disease of the skin and is of an inflammatory nature. It is more often known as dermatitis or inflammation of the skin.

Causes and Symptoms: Its symptoms are a scaly and fissured condition of the cuticle and a sticky watery discharge. There is itching or even pain. The condition is very important because it is said to embrace about one-half of all the cases of skin disease.

According to Ayurveda, eczema is a minor form of leprosy and is caused by the aggravation of *kapha* in addition to *vata* and *pitta*.

Medicines & Prescriptions: The following prescriptions are suggested, even though the medicines indicated for leprosy would undoubtedly help in ameliorating the condition of the patient.

1. *Udaya Bhaskara; Paribhadra Rasa; Chakramardabija Churna.*	120 mg *Udaya Bhaskara,* 240 mg *Paribhadra Rasa,* 240 mg *Chakramardabija Churna* to be taken thrice daily with *Khadiradirishta.*
2. *Root of Kasaundi.*	The root of *Kasaundi* should be ground and mixed with *Kanji* and applied on the affected part of the skin.

Home Remedies: Leaves of *amaltas* and their juice can also be rubbed over the affected parts.

Diet and Other Regimen: Since food is a major factor in the causation of eczema, one should particularly avoid eggs, seafood, and chocolates.

Soap should be used sparingly while taking a bath. Baby soap may be preferred. The patient should avoid using detergents with his hands.

Leucoderma *(Kilas)*

Leucoderma literally means 'white skin,' and is a condition in which there is a localised loss of pigmentation of the skin.

Causes and Symptoms: White patches appear on the skin. Ayurveda maintains that leucoderma is caused by some morbidity of the liver which results in a deficiency of *pitta.*

Medicines & Prescriptions: There are certain predisposing factors in leucoderma: persons suffering from chronic dysentery and other digestive disorders are more prone to it than others. If a patient of leucoderma is found to be suffering from digestive disorders, they should be treated first. *Kutaja (Holarrhena antidysenterica)* seems to be the drug of choice in this condition. Powder of the bark of the plant should be given in one teaspoonful doses thrice daily to correct the condition. *Arogyavardhini Vati* is another useful prescription: the normal dose is four tablets given thrice daily. *Bhallataka (Semecarpus* *anacardium*) is also helpful in treating this condition. A linctus prepared from the drug is given in one teaspoonful doses thrice daily. The side-effects that the drug is likely to have can be warded off by swallowing a little ghee or butter before ingesting the drug. It should be followed by a glass of milk.

The following prescriptions are specially recommended for *Kilas* patients:

1. *Rasa Manikya;* *Shashilekha Vati;* *Vakuchi Taila;* Honey.	60 mg *Rasa Manikya,* 240 mg *Shashilekha Vati,* and 4 ml each of *Vakuchi Taila* and honey to be taken thrice daily.
2. *Decoction of Khadira and Amla.*	One dose of 58 ml to be taken in the morning.
3. *Shweta Gunjadi Taila*	Should be applied on the affected parts.

Diet and Other Regimen: The patient should be kept on a salt-free diet as the absence of salt in the diet will speed up the recovery. Only rock salt is advised and that too in small quantities. Vegetables with a bitter taste like bitter gourd are beneficial.

Exposure to sun and heat should be avoided. The patient should avoid worry and mental strain. If he is costive, that condition should be ameliorated first before the regimen indicated above can help.

Psoriasis *(Eka Kushta)*

Psoriasis is a disease of the skin in which raised, rough, reddened areas appear, covered with fine silvery scales.

Causes and Symptoms: The eruption consists of a chronic inflammatory process in the true skin, the papillae of which become considerably lengthened and more vascular than usual. Changes in the cuticle also affect the epidermis. The condition generally appears for the first time around adolescence or early adult life. It is often a family disease occurring in different generations of one stock, and is often associated with gout or rheumatism. In some persons, psoriasis appears repeatedly at a particular season, especially in the spring and autumn, but it is not infectious.

The eruption almost always appears first round the back of the elbow and the front of the knees. It begins as small pimples, each covered with a white cap of scales, which enlarge in breadth till they form patches—two or three inches wide. At the same time, patches appear on other parts of the body, especially the scalp and the face.

Ayurveda believes that impurities in the blood associated with emotional factors are the cause of the disease.

Medicines & Prescriptions: *Kushta Rakshasa Taila* is the preparation of choice in treating this condition. It is for external application in case of itching in the affected parts. *Guggulu Tiktaka Ghrita* is given internally. It improves digestion and removes impurities from the blood. The patient should be on an empty stomach, and take one teaspoonful twice daily with a cup of hot milk. The dose is gradually increased to six teaspoonfuls. After some days when some improvement is visible, *Chandamrita* is given in a one grain dose with honey on empty stomach. Along with this, *Manjishtha* (decoction of the stem of the plant) should be administered in one ounce doses twice during the day.

Diet and Other Regimen: Spicy foods, curds, and salt should be avoided. If the patient cannot subsist on a salt-free diet, he may be permitted a little rock salt. Vegetables like drumsticks, bitter gourd, and flowers of the *neem* tree are helpful in dealing with this condition.

Clothes made of man-made fibres should not be worn by the patient. He should not scratch the affected parts but apply *Kushta Rakhasa Taila* over them.

Urticaria *(Shita Pitta)*

Urticaria or nettle-rash is a disorder of the skin. It is characterised by an eruption resembling the effect produced by the sting of a nettle.

Causes and Symptoms: Raised red and white patches occur in parts or over the whole surface of the body, and are accompanied by great itching and irritation.

Modern medicine believes allergy to be the causative factor of urticaria, but the real reason is the aggravation of *kapha* and *vayu* in conjunction with the vitiation of *pitta*. Sudden exposure to cold when the body is hot, as after exercise; infestation with parasites; and mental excitement are some of the causative factors.

Home Remedies: *Haridra* (*Curcuma longa*) or *haldi*, used in all Indian dishes, has long been recognised as the best remedy for urticaria. Regular use of it can prevent attacks of urticaria. A paste made of *haridra*, ground with a little water, may be given to the patient in two teaspoonful doses thrice a day. If the patient finds it unpalatable, it may be mixed with milk and sugar. The affected parts should be rubbed with mustard oil with which powdered rock salt has been mixed. The body should then be exposed to the sun and rubbed with a piece of copper.

Medicines & Prescriptions: An Ayurvedic preparation, *Haridra Khanda*, may be given in one teaspoonful doses thrice daily with lukewarm water. Another popular remedy is red ochre (*gairika*) or *geru*. *Kamadugdha Rasa*, which contains appreciable amounts of this substance, is given in five grain doses four times a day. Alternatively, *Suta Shekhara Rasa* and *Arogyavardhini Rasa* may be given in five grain doses thrice daily with honey. In case of constipation attending the complaint, a mild laxative may be given.

The following prescriptions are particularly recommended:

1. *Rasa Sindur; Haridra Khanda.*

   80 gm *Rasa Sindur* and 4 gm *Haridra Khanda* to be taken thrice daily with water.

2. *Powder of root of Arni.*

   3 gm of *Arni* to be taken with 12 gm of *ghee* twice daily.

3. A paste made of seeds of white mustard, turmeric, *Kooth*, seeds of *Chakramarda* and black sesame seeds should be massaged over the affected parts.

In case the patient suffers from intestinal worms, that condition should be treated first. If neglected, urticaria is likely to recur.

Diet and Other Regimen: A salt-free diet is recommended. Sour substances like curds should be avoided. All bitter substances and vegetables like drumsticks and bitter gourd are helpful. Onions and garlic should be taken in adequate quantities.

A food diary should be maintained indicating the relationship between a particular food and the appearance of symptoms.

Greying of Hair *(Palitya)*

Hair springs from the true skin, each hair having a root and a stem or shaft. The stem is generally rounded and varies greatly in thickness, while in the case of a curly hair, it is oval or flattened in section. The varying tint of the hair is due to pigment scattered in varying amounts throughout the hair. The rate of growth of hair is about 15 centimetres or 6 inches in a year, though in most persons, when the hair reaches a certain length, it ceases to grow at the root and is gradually pushed upwards till it falls out. It is then replaced by a new hair which develops from a fresh papilla.

Causes and Symptoms: An important part is played by the sebaceous glands which open into the follicles of the hair. Dryness of the hair in some persons is the result of malfunctioning of the sebaceous glands.

Hair has a tendency to lose its natural tint with age. A white hair is produced by the formation of numerous air spaces throughout the cells composing it. Greying of the hair in old age is natural but premature greying of the hair is a morbid condition. The causative factors include certain diseases like chronic colds, sinusitis, and a constitution given to excessive passion and worry. Persons who are given to washing their hair with hot water are more prone to suffer from premature greying of hair than others.

Medicines & Prescriptions: *Amrita* (*giloya*), *amla* and *gokhroo* taken in equal parts and mixed with honey should be taken in one teaspoonful doses thrice a day. Else, two parts of *Bhringraja,* one part of black sesame seeds, and one part of *amla* should be ground into powder. A teaspoonful of the powder should be taken with milk and sugar. But it has to be continued for some months before the effects are visible. *Swarnamakshika Bhasma* may be added in 240 mg doses with the powders in order to have early results. *Bhringaraja Taila* is the obvious remedy for external application. *Eladi Taila* can be used for massaging the head.

Old *mandur, amla, and japa* (*Hibiscus rosa sineusis*) flowers may be taken in equal quantities and ground into a paste. The paste should be applied over the head. After the paste dries, the hair should be washed with water in which *amla* has been soaked overnight.

Amla—2 parts, *harada*—2 parts, *bahera*—1 part, stone of mango—5 parts, and old *mandur*—2 ½ parts, should be ground together into a fine powder. A spoonful of the powder may be wetted with water in which *amla* has been soaked. The paste may be kept overnight in an iron vessel and applied to the hair in the morning. When it has dried, apply oil to the hair and then wash thoroughly.

Diet and Other Regimen: Fruits and vegetables should be taken in abundance to facilitate the supply of essential vitamins and minerals.

If the patient is suffering from allergic rhinitis, effort should be made to get it treated.

Baldness *(Khalitya)*
Baldness refers to a loss of hair, usually in the skull.

Causes and Symptoms: Baldness may be due to certain serious diseases like acute fevers, myxodema (a syndrome caused by hypothyroidism), syphilis, influenza, anaemia, and great anxiety or nervous shock. Premature baldness is generally considered to be hereditary and not much can be done except delaying the falling of the hair for some years through proper medication. Sometimes eczema of the scalp leads to rapid baldness.

Home Remedies: If the baldness is due to any of the serious diseases mentioned above, medication should start the moment the falling of the hair is noticed. A naturopathic remedy is the vigorous rubbing of the scalp with the fingers. This activates the sebaceous glands which nourish the hair and prevent its falling.

Medicines & Prescriptions: The administration of drugs indicated for premature greying of hair should help in the cases of baldness also, but recourse to medication has to be taken in the earlier stages. If all the hair has fallen out and the follicles have closed, nothing much can be done. Those who attach a lot of cosmetic value to their hair may wear a wig.

Note: Diet and other regimen to be followed should also be the same as for premature greying, but these can only be effective in the early stages of baldness.

Diseases of the Eyes, Ears, Teeth & Gums

तथा ऋतूनां च विपर्ययेण क्लेशाभिघातादतिमैथुनाच्च ।
बाष्पग्रहात् सूक्ष्मनिरीक्षणाच्च नेत्रे विकारान् जनयन्ति दोषाः ॥

Not observing the advisable seasonal regimen, heat, exacerbation of grief, injury, excessive sexual intercourse, suppression of tears and straining the eyes, leads to vitiation of Vayu and that leads to many diseases of the eye.

BHOJARATNAKAR

CARE OF the eyes, ears, teeth, and gums is vital for the well-being of an individual. Any damage to these parts of the body, particularly, the eyes and the ears can seriously handicap a person's functioning.

Diseases of the Eye

The organs of sight—the eyes—are, perhaps, the most delicate part of the body. They are set in a deep four-sided cavity in the skull called the orbit. The edges of this are so prominent, especially above and to the inner side, that a flat object resting on them does not touch the eyeball and, therefore, the eye is very seldom injured by a blow. But the delicacy of structure of the eye renders any disorder of this organ highly important. Many of the disorders of the eye can be cured to a limited extent, and in some cases, surgical interference is needed, as in the case of opacity of the cornea, known as cataract. But if opacity is noticed in the earlier stages and proper steps are taken in time, the development of the cataract can be delayed for a long time.

Sushruta has recognised seventy-six distinct disorders of the eye; some of the old masters have counted upto seventy-eight diseases which afflict the eye. Of these, the most serious is the opacity of the cornea which results in dimness of sight and sometimes total loss of it, if glaucoma is at the root of the opacity.

Cataract *(Timira* or *Lin Ganasha)*

When the lens of the eye loses its transparency, the vision is more or less completely blocked. This condition is known as cataract.

Causes and Symptoms: The most common form of cataract is the senile cataract which begins at about the age of fifty in eyes which may have been perfectly healthy. The disorder is also one of the offshoots of diabetes. It may also be the result of any injury to the eye or its exposure to intense heat, as in the case of glass workers. Irradiation cataract can be caused by X-rays, radium, or nuclear energy. The passage of electric current through the body may, in some cases, be followed by the development of what is known as electric cataract.

The first symptom of cataract is the appearance of floating specks in the vision. Bright objects seem to be multiplied, especially bright lights at a distance in the dark. A moderate degree of short-sightedness may come in, which is relieved for a time by spectacles. Gradually, increasing blindness is the most apparent symptom. In the early stages, the person may be less blind in the dusk than in bright light, because only the centre of the lens is affected, and a clear part round the edge permits the light to reach the inner eye.

Ayurveda attributes cataract to the aggravation of *vayu,* which dries up the eyeball, making it opaque.

Medicines & Prescriptions: The first thing in dealing with a case of cataract is to reduce the aggravation of *vayu*, for which *ghee* in its medicated form is the best remedy. *Mahatriphala Ghrita* is the supreme remedy for cataract. It has to be remembered, however, that it is efficacious only in the preliminary stages of the disease when the opacity of the lens is just beginning to develop. The medicated *ghee* should

102

be given to the patient in two teaspoonful doses twice daily. It should be mixed with warm milk.

Chandrodaya Vati rubbed into a paste with human breast milk or honey should be applied to the eyes; it is a mild irritant but it promotes blood circulation and lacrimation (tears) in the eyes and hence, provides nourishment to the tissues of the eye. *Triphala* water—water in which the three myrobalans, *harada*, *bahera*, and *amla* have been soaked overnight—should be used for washing the eyes and also taken internally. This will also keep the patient free from constipation which interferes with the treatment of cataract.

Diet and Other Regimen: Cow's milk and its products are extremely useful for a person suffering from cataract. Vegetables like fenugreek, spinach, drumsticks, lady's fingers; and fruits like banana, grapes, pomegranate, apples, and oranges are recommended. Pungent, bitter, and sour foodstuffs should be avoided. The patient should be permitted only rock salt and that too in small quantities.

The patient should avoid exposure to heat and the sun. Excessive mental strain or emotional strain should be avoided as it leads to aggravation of *vayu* and *pitta*, which lead to the disorder in the first place.

Myopia *(Dristi Dosha)*

Myopia or short-sight is a condition in which, owing to the lens of the eye being too highly convex or the ball of the eye being too long, rays of light are brought to a focus before they reach the retina, and so form circles of diffused light upon it. It is the opposite of hypermetropia or long vision.

Causes and Symptoms: Myopia generally occurs in the young; the patient experiences difficulty in seeing far- off objects. Spectacles with concave lenses of the required curvature may help in correcting the vision, but the defect continues to increase with age, and the patient of this type of progressive myopia has to continue to change the lenses of his spectacles.

Nervous debility and susceptibility to cold and constipation are, according to Ayurveda, the predisposing factors responsible for myopia. It begins with blurred vision, particularly with regard to objects at a distance and, later, leads to an inability to recognise persons unless they are standing next to the sufferer. The blackboard and the screen in a motion picture house may become blurred for the viewer. The eyes may water due to strain, and an itch and a sensation of heaviness and burning may be experienced in the eyes. An offshoot of the malady may be headaches, and loss of or disturbance in sleep.

Medicines & Prescriptions: The first requirement before any cure of myopia can be undertaken is to rid the patient of cold and constipation. Any tendency towards constipation is likely to interfere with the course of the treatment. *Triphala* should be administered to deal with these ailments. *Triphala* water should be drunk and also used for washing the eyes thoroughly. Four ounces of decoction of *triphala* should be taken to relieve the constipation and the dose may have to be regulated according to the severity of the constipation. Washing with *triphala* water and taking it internally may have to be continued for three to four months to deal with the condition. The other medicine of choice for myopia is *Yashthi Madhu (Glycyrrhiza glabra)*. The powder of the root of the plant is given in a half teaspoonful dose, mixed with a quarter spoon of pure *ghee* and half teaspoon of honey. The dose is to be given twice daily on an empty stomach.

If myopia is of nervous origin, namely, if it has been caused by nervous debility, *Saptamrita Lauha* is the obvious remedy. A teaspoonful of this medicine is given twice daily with milk. In case of constipation, the obvious remedy is *Mahatriphala Ghrita*, the dose of which may be increased to three teaspoonfuls twice daily with milk. Cold and nasal congestion may be dealt with by dropping five to six drops of *Shadbindu Taila* into each nostril.

Diet and Other Regimen: Pungent and sour foods are to be avoided as are those which may exacerbate costiveness. Fried things should be prohibited, though *ghee* made from cow's milk may be used in moderate quantities.

The patient is advised to avoid eye strain. Continuous reading is not helpful—after a few pages of reading, the patient should rest his eyes for some minutes. Work demanding concentration of eyesight, as in needlework; and reading and writing at night should not be permitted. Walking barefoot on dew-covered grass and long walks in the morning are helpful. One should not read while lying in bed.

Conjunctivitis *(Abhishyanda)*

Conjunctivitis is an inflammation of the conjunctiva or mucous membrane connecting the inner eyelid and eyeball. It is a very common eye affection. Though not serious in itself, it may give rise to complications such as the ulceration of the cornea.

Causes and Symptoms: A chronic state of redness of the eye is common among people whose eyes are much exposed to irritation from dust, smoke, cold winds, and the like. Strain on the eyes because of errors of refraction (where the patient needs glasses in order to have a normal vision) may cause the eye to appear red, as a cold in the head would lead to congestion of the conjunctiva.

The most characteristic sign of conjunctivitis is that the affected eye becomes red or bloodshot because of the dilatation of the numerous vessels which ramify over the conjunctival surface. The swelling of the conjunctiva in severe cases may be marked, and a thickened fold may form round the edge of the cornea. Subjective symptoms vary greatly; in some cases, only a feeling of having sand in the eyes is experienced, whereas in others, there is acute pain. Photophobia or dread of light is a common symptom. There is discharge of mucous from the eyes which may deteriorate into pus. Usually both the eyes are affected even though the trouble starts in one eye.

In addition to simple acute conjunctivitis, there are other more serious varieties: ophthalmia of the newborn which may attack infants a few days after they are born; trachoma or granular conjunctivitis which is a persistent and severe form of the disease prevalent in Asia and other countries in the East; follicular conjunctivitis; and phlectenular conjunctivitis, which usually attacks weak, ill-nourished children.

Home Remedies: The very first step in the treatment of conjunctivitis is to keep the eyes clean. Fomentation and cleaning with hot water in which borax (*suhaga*) has been dissolved is useful in giving relief and also in keeping the eyes clean. A paste made of candied sugar, alum, and rock salt in quantities of 3 gm each; 6 gm *rasaut;* and 117 ml rose water should be used as eye drops. Five to six minims (drops) of the mixture should be put into the eyes three to four times in the day. Four grams each of alua, large *harada* (*Haridra longa*), alum roasted over a hot plate, and 1 gm of opium should be ground together with a little water to form a paste which should be applied over the eyelids.

Medicines & Prescriptions: In addition to the above, 240 ml of *Netrashni Rasa* should be taken with hot water twice daily. In case conjunctivitis has become chronic, *Rasanjanadi Rasakriya* should be used as collyrium. Along with this, 250 mg roasted alum should be mixed with 30 ml of *triphala* decoction and used as eye drops. Eight drops of the mixture should be dropped into the eyes five to six times in the day. Three doses of *Netrashni Rasa* should be given with 10 gms of *Mahatriphaladi Ghrita* thrice—before, during, and after meals.

Diet and Other Regimen: Sour substances should be avoided.

The patient should avoid eye strain. Dark goggles may be worn during the day. The bowels should not be allowed to become costive. Mild laxatives may be taken recourse to if constipation develops.

Trachoma (*Pothaki*)

Trachoma or granular conjunctivitis is a chronic and severe form of conjunctivitis, and is the greatest single cause of serious and progressive loss of sight. It is estimated that there are more than 400 million people in the world suffering from this disease and it has been a source of worry for the World Health Organisation and the health authorities of the various countries of the world.

Causes and Symptoms: Modern medicine believes that trachoma is of viral origin and claims to have separated the virus responsible for it.

Trachoma is characterised by the appearance of nodules—pale in colour, and often compared to boiled sago grains—situated on the conjunctival lining of the lids. Very often, the upper half of the cornea becomes covered with a hazy film containing a network of superficial blood vessels. In the later stages of the disease, there is much scarring and shrinking of the conjunctiva, and the lids are apt to be torn inwards, thereby causing the lashes to rub on the cornea. Loss of transparency of the cornea and consequent dimness of vision are, therefore, frequent results of this disease. A very large number of cases of blindness can be traced to chronic trachoma.

Medicines & Prescriptions: *Lekhyanjana*—a compound of *kashis*, rock salt, *trikatu,* and calx of horn—taken in equal quantities should be used for the eyes. Alternatively, *Chandrodaya Vati*, *Chandraprabha Vati*, and *Churnanjana* should be ground with honey and used as collyrium. The eyes should be washed with warm water in which borax has been dissolved.

Home Remedies: Six grams of alum, 1 gm of *tutia*, and 120 ml of rose water should be made into a mixture and used as eye drops. Pure mustard oil, used as eye drops, is also helpful in this condition.

Diet and Other Regimen: The same dietary regimen is to be followed as in the case of conjunctivitis.

Eyes should be protected from bright light and wearing of dark goggles is recommended. Strain to the eyes should be avoided.

Diseases of the Ear

The organ of hearing—the ear—has two functions. The more obvious, of course, is that of the sense of hearing, but the other is the sense of equilibration and of motion. The ear is divided into three parts: the external ear; the middle ear, separated from the former by the tympanic membranes and from the internal ear by two other membranes, but communicating with the throat by the Eustachian tube; and the internal ear comprising the complicated labyrinth from which the auditory nerve runs into the brain.

Troubles connected with the ear should, whenever possible, be treated early, both on account of this organ's importance, and because, owing to its delicacy and inaccessibility, little can be done for unpleasant symptoms like deafness and ringing due to advanced disease.

Earache *(Kaan Ka Dard)*

A common auditory affliction is an ache in the ear. This condition should be treated in consultation with a physician.

Causes and Symptoms: Earache may be due to acute inflammation in the middle ear, but may also be due to chronic inflammation, boils, eczema, wax, or neuralgia affecting the outer ear. Pain in this region may also be due to decay in a tooth.

Home Remedies: The treatment varies, of course, according to the cause of the ache, but the pain is generally removed by application of heat. In some cases, heated mustard oil might suffice. But if a pod of garlic is burnt in a spoonful of any edible oil, allowed to cool sufficiently, and then dropped into the affected ear and plugged with a piece of cotton, the pain will subside. Saline gargles are recommended twice daily.

Ringing in the Ear or Tinnitus

Ringing is a noise heard in the ear without any external cause.

Causes and Symptoms: Tinnitus may take various forms, but is, in general, accompanied by catarrh of some part of the ear. Pulsating or throbbing in the ear is sometimes due to bloodlessness, or to large doses of quinine or some other allopathic medicine.

Medicines & Prescriptions: This condition is difficult to treat. However, if the real cause can be detected and treated, the problem is likely to be remedied.

Discharge from the Ear *(Putikama)*

The most serious of ear ailments is, of course, a discharge from the ear which may arise in the external ear.

Causes and Symptoms: A discharge from the ear may be a result of eczema, boils, or irritation caused by a plug of wax or foreign body. But in the absence of these, in a great majority of cases, it is a result of a chronic suppuration in a the middle ear through a perforation of the drum. The suppuration may begin with an acute inflammation of the middle ear arising in the course of a 'cold in the head'; or may result from scarlet fever or measles; or may be due to disease of the bone in or around the ear; or may simply have a slow onset, without any apparent cause in weak persons, especially in children. The discharge may be thick and yellowish in cases which are fairly acute, or thin and watery in cases which are improving. If the suppuration continues without proper treatment for any length of time, it may result in deafness. If deafness begins as a concomitant of suppuration, it might be due to an abscess in the region of the ear, or even in the skull.

Vitiation of *kapha*, according to Ayurveda, is the cause of suppuration of the ear or *putikarna*.

Medicines & Prescriptions: *Sarivadi Vati* is a cardinal remedy for the condition described above. The adult dose is one pill given thrice a day with honey. The preparation for external application is *Nirgundi* (*Viteh negundi*); the juice of the plant is boiled with mustard oil and the medicated oil is used as ear drops. Another medicine for external application is *Bilva* (*Aegle marmelos);* the paste of the root of the plant is boiled with mustard oil.

Diet and Other Regimen: Foods which tend to vitiate or aggravate *kapha* like curds, bananas, guavas, and sour fruits should be avoided. Garlic, ginger, and onions should be taken in adequate quantities.

Exposure to cold and wind is to be avoided.

Disorders of the Teeth and Gums

Teeth are hard organs developed in connection with the mucous membrane of the mouth and implanted in the jaw bones. In man they serve for biting and grinding the food, as well as aiding in speech. In many animals, they are adapted as weapons.

Considering the fact that the teeth are highly sensitive, that any interference with their use causes marked disturbance of digestion, and that good teeth form a highly aesthetic feature, disorders of these structures are of great importance. Ayurveda recognises as many as fifteen diseases of the gums, including gum boils and spongy gums, but the most serious disorder is that of pyorrhoea.

Pyorrhoea *(Dantaveshta* or *Putidanta)*

Pyorrhoea is a condition characterised in the final stages by the promotion of pockets of purulent material around the teeth and loosening of the affected teeth.

Causes and Symptoms: The prevalent opinion among allopaths is that the lack of roughage in the diet and inadequate care of the teeth is the causative factor in pyorrhoea. These two factors lead to stagnation of food between the teeth and excessive formation of tartar, which, in turn, leads to proliferation of bacteria. It leads to an unpleasant taste in the mouth and a foul smell. Ulceration of gums and chronic inflammatory changes are the usual concomitants of this disease.

Ayurveda recognises the absence of oral hygiene as a causative factor in pyorrhoea, but the real cause is digestive disorders, because it is generally those with a costive constitution and a bad digestion who fall prey to pyorrhoea.

Home Remedies: The first step in the direction of treatment is oral hygiene. It is better to brush one's teeth with a six-inch twig of the *neem* tree or the banyan tree *(Ficus bengalensis)*. The latex or milk of the prop root inhibits the formation of pus because of its antiseptic qualities. Being astringent, it also stops bleeding from the gums.

Medicines & Prescriptions: For constipation, a decoction of *triphala* is the best remedy and must be taken recourse to if the patient suffers from it. The powders of the bark of *bakula* (*Mimusops elengi*) and *babula* (*Acacia arabica*) should be used as tooth powders. The well-known Ayurvedic preparation *Dashana Sanskara Churna*, for use as tooth powder, is of great efficacy in preventing any further deterioration in the condition of a patient of pyorrhoea. Hot water mixed with borax should be used for gargles. The gums should be rubbed with *Bhadramustadi Gutika.*

Diet and Other Regimen: The patient is advised to increase intake of fruits and vegetables to increase the input of vitamins and minerals.

The patient should gargle with alum regularly.

Toothache *(Daant Ka Dard)*

Toothache can be due to many causes, most of which pertain to local infections.

Home Remedies: Minor ailments like toothache can be handled by applying clove oil to the area of pain.

Medicines & Prescriptions: In case of decay or crumbling of a tooth, latex of the *madar* plant should be used; it kills the organisms which produce the caries.

Kalka Churna mixed with honey and applied to the throat in throat affections, or kept in the mouth in diseases of the mouth, helps cure many diseases of the teeth and the mouth. Another beneficial preparation in these conditions is *Peetaka Churna* mixed with honey and *ghee.* Swarjika yoga is a well-known remedy for toothache.

Diet and Other Regimen: As in all other cases of illness, diet is of the most vital importance in dental disorders. Sticky substances which may adhere to the teeth should be avoided, as also sugar and other sweets. Fruits like guavas, pomegranates, oranges, and other fruits of the citrus family are beneficial as they contain Vitamin C which strengthens the gums. *Amla,* it must be remembered, contains the largest amount of Vitamin C and is cheap to boot. It must form a part of the diet of a victim of dental disorders, whether in raw form or cooked as a vegetable.

The mouth should be rinsed after each meal.

Diseases of the Liver & the Cardio-vascular System

प्रतिष्ठार्थं हि भावानामेषां हृदयमिष्यते ।
गोपानसी नामागारकर्णिकेवार्थचिन्तकैः ॥

As the central girder supports the wood or bamboo framework of thatch, so the heart represents the substratum of all the organs of the body. Even a small injury to the heart results in fainting.

CHARAKA SAMHITA

THE NUTRITION that the human body assimilates through the ingestion of food is turned into blood which travels through the different organs. Blood is being constantly manufactured, purified, and replaced. In a normal, healthy human body, the amount of blood is nine per cent of the body weight.

Blood (*Ahara Rasa*)

Its constituents—the red and white corpuscles and platelets—have their own allotted functions to perform. The red corpuscles act as oxygen carriers; the white corpuscles act as guards who fight infection; and the platelets help in the coagulation of the vital fluid in cases of injury. The fluid, the main constituent of blood, carries the various salts and proteins which nourish the tissues. Blood restores the tissues and replaces the energy that we lose through the use of our body. It journeys downwards from the heart which pushes it through the body. It carries the various waste products like carbonic acid gas to be exhaled by the lungs, and the urea and the salts

112

to be removed by the kidneys. Blood forms a general medium of communication between the organs that are chemically interdependent: it carries to the stomach, the materials for the gastric juice; to the muscles, the ferments formed in the pancreas; and it absorbs secretions needed for the general purposes of the body, like those of the thyroid gland and the suprarenal glands.

According to Ayurveda, however, blood is formed from *ahara rasa* which is produced as a result of the assimilation of food. *Ahara rasa* is driven by *prana vayu* through the vessels to the heart, and from there, carried to the different parts of the body. From the *ahara rasa* are produced the different *dhatus* of the body, the first of them being the *rasa dhatu*, the raw material of blood.

The heart, according to the *Kedari Kulya Nyaya* (irrigation channel analogy), is like a tank; the *ahara rasa* like the water; the *dhamanis* (blood vessels) like the water channels. The *ahara rasa* is not returned to the heart, according to this theory. Instead, *fresh rasa* is manufactured from the food that is digested.

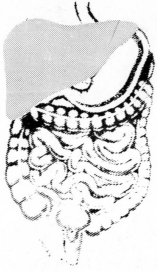

Liver and G.I. Tract
113

We shall deal first with the primary organ, the liver, which is the storehouse of nourishment.

Functions of the Liver

The liver is a large chemical factory; the heat produced by the chemical changes taking place in it contributes greatly to the general warming of the body. The liver secretes bile, which comprises salts and pigments, and aids the digestion of fats. It stores the substance necessary for the proper functioning of the bone marrow which manufactures red blood corpuscles. It also manufactures the fibrinogen of the blood, stores iron and copper, and detoxicates the noxious products which are made in the intestines and absorbed into the blood. It stores carbohydrates in the form of glycogen.

The liver is one of the largest organs in the body and one of the five major organs which are vital to life. A malfunctioning of the liver may not become apparent immediately, unless, of course, the blood flow through it is impeded or the bile ducts are obstructed. Nor does it recover quickly once it suffers from a disorder.

Cirrhosis of the Liver *(Yakrit Vriddhi)*

Cirrhosis of the liver is a chronic disease characterised by progressive destruction and scarring of liver cells. The tissues are replaced by fibrous tissues similar to scar tissues.

Causes and Symptoms: The colour of the organ turns from red to yellow and it contracts. There is a tendency for the body to swell up. Cirrhosis of the liver is of many types. When it develops among children, it is generally due to a faulty diet and is known as infantile cirrhosis. In adults, it is generally the result of excessive intake of alcohol.

Cirrhosis of the liver manifests itself in the congestion of the organ, and that results in loss of appetite. Diarrhoea and flatulence may follow, and then pain in the region of the liver is noticed. Pressure of the expanding liver on the diaphragm and the muscular wall separating the lungs and the heart from the other organs in the abdomen may cause difficulty in breathing, along with a cough.

114

The liver helps to neutralize the toxic effects of substances ingested, and if such substances are taken in excess or are faulty, it may fail to meet the demands made on it. The first thing that should be done before medication is started in a case of cirrhosis of the liver is to ban all intoxicating substances like tea, coffee, tobacco, and alcohol.

Medicines & Prescriptions: The best remedy for cirrhosis of the liver is *Bhringaraja* (*Eclipta alba*), a small herb which grows in marshy lands. The juice of the leaves, flowers, stems, and roots of the plant is administered in doses of one teaspoonful thrice daily in the case of infantile cirrhosis. The juice should be mixed with honey to offset its bitter and astringent taste.

Katuki (*Picrorrhiza kurroa*) is the drug of choice for cirrhosis among adults. The root of the herb which grows at high altitudes is given in powdered form. One teaspoonful of the powder, mixed with an equal amount of honey, is administered thrice daily. In case of attendant constipation, the dose should be increased to double and be given with a cup of warm water three to four times a day. It stimulates the liver to produce more bile, the excretion of which relieves congestion of the liver; and the tissues which have become defunct start functioning again. An Ayurvedic medicine, *Aarogyavardhani*, a compound of *katuki* and calx of copper, can be administered with advantage in cirrhosis of the liver. It has the property of reviving the cells which have become atrophied. A 250 mg tablet of this medicine is available, and two to four tablets should be given thrice during the day with a cupful of warm water.

Drugs prescribed for jaundice or hepatitis (*kamala* in Ayurveda) are also helpful in a case of cirrhosis of the liver as they strengthen the liver.

Diet and Other Regimen: The main thing to be noted, however, is that the diet is more important than any medication in cases of diseases of the liver. All fatty substances and hard-to-digest foods should be banned. Skimmed milk or goat's milk, juice of sugarcane, buttermilk instead of curds, and garlic should be prescribed. In case there is accumulation of fluids in the region of the abdomen (dropsy), a salt-free diet should be given to the patient.

Constipation should not be allowed to develop at any cost even if it means a daily purgative or an enema. If the patient feels lost without intake of salt, he may be permitted to use a little rock salt—marine salt is like poison in ailments of the liver.

In addition, the patient should be advised to take complete rest. He should not sleep during the day, or ride a vehicle which might jerk the whole body, or take any violent exercise. The only exertion permitted is walking over flat, even ground to avoid shaking the body.

Jaundice *(Kamala)*

Jaundice or *kamala* is a condition in which there is discoloration of the skin because of deposition of bile pigment in its deeper layers.

Causes and Symptoms: Jaundice may be caused by inflammation of the liver which is known as hepatitis, an infection, or an obstruction of the bile ducts due to cirrhosis. It can also be caused by ingestion of certain poisonous substances, the morbidity of which the liver is unable to deal with. Whatever the technical name, many diseases of the liver result in jaundice.

The yellow colour first appears in the white of the eyes and then spreads to the whole skin. Excess of bile pigment—*pitta*—circulating in the blood gives the skin its yellow colour. The bile does not go into the intestine as it should, and so, the stools of the jaundiced patient lose their typical brownish colour, and in severe cases, are almost whitish. There is loss of appetite and impairment of digestion. The liver is unable to digest fat and there may be a sense of fullness at the time. Nausea may also be present in certain cases because of defective digestion. If the liver is inflamed, there is also pain in the region of the organ and it is tender to touch.

Medicines & Prescriptions: The treatment of jaundice must start with purgation. The basic theory is that no burden be placed on the liver and for that, a daily purgative (allopaths recommend a saline purgative) is recommended. A diuretic may also be administered to encourage the flow of urine which will expel most of the bile from the system.

Trivari (Operculina turpenthum) and *katuki* (mentioned earlier while dealing with cirrhosis of the liver) are the two major drugs with which the treatment of jaundice should start. One to two teaspoonfuls of the powder of the drugs may be administered with hot water twice daily. A well-known combination of drugs used by Ayurveda for the treatment of jaundice is *Avipattikar Churna* and *Arogyavardhini Vati*. The *Churna* should be given in one teaspoonful doses twice a day with hot water. *Arogyavardhini Vati* is available in 250 mg strength, and two tablets should be given thrice daily with hot water or with honey. Other drugs used in the treatment of jaundice are: *Vasaka (Adhatoda vasica)*, *Kakamachi (Solanum nigrum)*, and *triphala* (the three myrobalans). Any or all the above drugs may be prescribed depending upon the condition of the patient.

Home Remedies: A popular method to encourage the flow of copious urine in a patient suffering from jaundice is to soak a piece of tender bark of the *peepul* tree (2"×1"×6") in water overnight and drink the water in the morning.

Diet and Other Regimen: Sweet substances and liquids like sugarcane juice, fruit juice, and dry grapes should form the mainstay of the patient's diet. Spices, fats, alcohol, and tobacco are contraindicated. Buttermilk is the best drink for a patient suffering from jaundice.

The patient is advised complete rest.

Anaemia *(Pandu Roga)*

Anaemia is the lack of red blood corpuscles and haemoglobin in the blood.

Causes and Symptoms: Anaemia may be caused by loss of blood through excessive menstruation, injury, childbirth, bleeding from the gastro-intestinal tract, certain diseases like purpura and haemophilia which are characterised by bleeding; defective blood formation because of infections, toxins, and drugs; inadequate intake of iron; and defective absorption of substances in the diet which enrich the blood. Some anaemias are due to a combination of more than one of the causes enumerated above.

The most striking symptom of anaemia is the pallor of the skin, hence the Ayurvedic name, *Pandu Roga*. The best guide, however, is the colour of the internal lining of the eyelid. There is weakness and giddiness, the breathing is shallow, the pulse rapid, and the blood pressure low. In severe cases, the tongue is often sore and the nails of the fingers brittle and concave instead of being convex. If the disease is ignored, it may turn into pernicious anaemia which is more difficult to cure. In some severe cases, the patient may have to be given a blood transfusion to make up the loss of blood, as happens in traumas like severe haemorrhage due to injury or bursting of an ulcer in the abdominal region.

Medicines & Prescriptions: Before treatment can be started, the exact cause of the malady should be ascertained. If it is of a mild nature and has been caused by insufficient nutrition, massive doses of the substances lacking could cure it. But if it is due to malfunctioning of the liver, the stomach, or the bone marrow, *Punarnavadi Mandura* or *Punarnava Mandura* are the medicines of choice. One gram of *Mandura* should be given with honey four times a day. For children, the dose can be suitably reduced. The main ingredient of the drug is *punarnava* (*Boerhaavia diffusa*) which has rejuvenating qualities. If given to healthy persons, it acts as an elixir.

Vyoshadi Ghrita, *Phaltrikadi Kashaya*, *Pandu Panchanana Rasa* and *Lauhasava* are some of the other drugs and standard Ayurvedic preparations useful in anaemia.

Home Remedies: Fresh liver of goat—lightly cooked, and fresh blood of goat or rabbit can immediately help fight the severity of anaemia.

Diet and Other Regimen: Fruit juice, milk, meat soup, green vegetables, and light foods free from fats and sour substances are recommended for a patient suffering from anaemia. Sweet mango is like nectar for such a patient.

If the patient is constipated, purgatives are indicated because anaemia is born of *pitta* which can be corrected through purgation. *Triphala* water (the three myrobalans soaked in water) is the best remedy for such constipation.

Leukaemia *(Vatolvana Sannipataja Pandu Roga)*

Leukaemia, commonly known as cancer of the blood, is a disease, usually of chronic type, in which the number of white corpuscles of the blood is permanently increased. In many ways, it resembles a form of malignant disease.

Causes and Symptoms: In cases of acute leukaemia, the patient shows pallor, occasional purpuric rash, and enlargement of the lymphatic glands and spleen. The temperature rises and the condition is liable to be mistaken for general TB. In cases of chronic leukaemia, the onset is gradual, and the usual symptoms are either swelling of the abdomen or shortness of breath due to painless enlargement of the spleen, or of the glands in the neck and armpits. Symptoms of anaemia such as a pale pallor of the skin and palpitations are present. There may also be occasional haemorrhages from the nose, stomach, gums, or bowels. There is dropsy of the feet, diarrhoea, and also a slight degree of fever. The life expectancy of the patient is not more than a few years if the disease is not treated in time.

Ayurveda believes that leukaemia is caused by a vitiation of all the three *doshas,* namely, *vata, pitta,* and *kapha,* and seeks to cure it with drugs which restore the balance of the three.

Medicines & Prescriptions: For acute cases of leukaemia, the following prescription is recommended:

Bajra Bhasma	5.8 mg of *Bajra Bhasma,*
(calx of diamond);	60 mg of *Muktapishtha,*
Muktapishtha;	and 120 mg of
Pandupanchanan Rasa.	*Pandupanchanan Rasa* to be taken thrice daily.

In chronic cases of leukaemia, the following prescription is recommended:

Bajra Bhasma; *Yakritaplihodarariloha Rasa;* *Pandupanchanan Rasa.*	5.8 mg of *Bajra Bhasma,* and 120 mg each of *Yakritaplihodarariloha Rasa* and *Pandupanchanan Rasa* to be taken thrice daily.

Other drugs recommended in leukaemia are: *Vishadi Churna, Davyardileha, Chandrasuryatmak Rasa, Trailokyasundar.*

Periodic transfusions of blood may also be necessary in chronic cases of leukaemia.

Home Remedies: In addition to the above, a decoction of fresh liver juice and turmeric should be given. Fresh blood of goat and rabbit, taken in doses of 50 to 100 ml, is also helpful in acute cases.

Diet and Other Regimen: The patient suffering from leukaemia should be advised to eat old rice and oats, *moong dal*, vegetables like raw banana, gourds, spinach, raw papaya, radish, and onions; *amla*, figs, oranges, apples and grapes; meats like fresh liver grilled over an open fire, and meat soups; butter, buttermilk, and *ghee*.

Care should be taken that no injury is caused to any part of the body, as this may lead to excessive bleeding.

Haemorrhage (*Rakta Pitta*)

Haemorrhage means any escape of blood from the vessels which normally carry it.

Causes and Symptoms: A haemorrhage may be external, as in the case of an injury. It may also be internal, due to an injury sustained in an accident by a blow, as in a fight; due to the bursting of an ulcer in the stomach; or due to some other disorder of an internal organ. Arterial haemorrhage is more serious than venous: the blood from an artery is bright in colour and comes out in spurts corresponding to the heartbeat. The haemorrhage from a vein is slow and the blood, dark in colour. In the case of a large artery being involved as the femoral artery, the blood loss is so rapid and copious that unless treated in time, the patient may not have long to live. Small arteries, when cut, may automatically close after some time due to their tendency to retract into the surrounding tissues, but surgical interference is necessary in the case of large arteries being torn. A venous haemorrhage can be controlled by applying pressure to the affected area. In serious cases of blood loss, the patient may have to be hospitalised for blood transfusion to make up the loss of the vital fluid.

Haemorrhage may be in the form of haematemesis (vomiting of blood) or sudden discharge of blood from other orifices of the body, as in piles. Ayurvedic theory ascribes bleeding to *Rakta Pitta* or the vitiation of the *pitta* in the blood. That is why Ayurvedic practitioners do not immediately stop the bleeding in a healthy individual. It is the vitiated blood, full of toxins, which is the first to come out of the body in a case of haemorrhage. This should be allowed to flow for some time, keeping in mind, of course, the patient's physique. If the bleeding is checked immediately, it may give rise to other disorders such as fainting, fever, loss of appetite, and other ailments.

Home Remedies: In haematemesis, the drug of choice is *amla* (*Emblica officinalis*); juice of this fruit should be given in 50 ml doses thrice a day. Similarly, juice of *kushmanda* (*Benincasa hispida*) could be administered in 50 ml doses thrice daily. Alternatively, *Pravala Pishthi* may be administered in 1 gm doses thrice in the day. For checking the bleeding, iced or refrigerated water should be given.

Medicines & Prescriptions: In other cases of *Rakta Pitta*, *Raktapittakulakand Rasa* is a better remedy; it should be given in doses of 250 mg to 1 gm thrice daily. *Pittantaka Rasa*, *Chandrakala Rasa*, *Ushirasava*, and *Mahapittantaka Rasa* are some of the other Ayurvedic remedies useful for this condition.

In case of internal haemorrhages, the patient should be warned to learn to recognise the signs of excessive bleeding. They are: palpitations, a sense of uneasiness, weakness, and profuse sweating. If the blood pressure of the patient has fallen considerably and continues to fall, immediate recourse to blood transfusion must be taken to save his life.

Diet and Other Regimen: A strict regimen of diet and abstinence from foodstuffs which may aggravate *pitta* is as important as the drugs prescribed above. Fruits like *amla*, dates, pomegranate, oranges, apples, bananas, grapes and dried grapes; juice of sugarcane, and water of coconut; and non-irritating vegetables are recommended.

The patient is advised to take complete rest and stay in cool surroundings; in summer, he should migrate to a cold climate.

Hypertension or High Blood Pressure *(Rakta Vata)*

Hypertension (*Rakta Vata*) or high blood pressure is a disorder characterised by more than normal pressure at which the blood is being pumped by the heart. The main function of the heart is to pump blood into the arteries and to receive the blood that comes back to it, after having completed a circuit of the whole body within fifteen seconds. With each beat of the heart, the blood is pumped out to the various organs through the arteries. When there is a disorder of the arteries such as arteriosclerosis (hardening of the arteries or deposition of fat in their insides), they are unable to contain the amount of blood that is necessary for a normal functioning of its circulation throughout the body, with the result that the heart is strained and works overtime to maintain the required amount of blood. In that process, it pumps with greater vigour and what is known as 'high' pressure of the blood is caused.

Causes and Symptoms: The normal pressure in a healthy adult is generally taken to be about 140 to 150 mm of mercury (systolic) and 80 mm (diastolic). Depending upon individual constitutions, any variation from the normal gives rise to symptoms like a headache, a sensation of ringing in the ears, pressure in the frontal region of the head, palpitations, and a general feeling of unease. Hypertension may be categorised as being either essential or functional. It may be caused in the latter case as a result of malfunctioning of the kidneys, giving rise to a high urea content in the blood. Stress or anxiety may be the other causes of functional hypertension.

According to Ayurveda, however, hypertension is a result of vitiation of *vayu*. Excessive use of alcohol and other intoxicants; salt; lack of exercise, leading to continuous inactivity of the heart muscle under conditions of stress—are all reasons for hypertension.

The cardinal symptoms of hypertension are: inability to sleep well, palpitations, giddiness, weakness, and impairment of digestion. If the disorder becomes chronic due to carelessness or lack of proper medication, the capillaries supplying blood to the retina may become disordered and there may be impairment of vision. If the blood supply to the brain fails as a complication of high blood pressure, the patient may fall victim to a stroke. There may be cerebral haemorrhage, resulting in paralysis or even death.

Home Remedies: The treatment of hypertension must start with a proper diagnosis of its origin. If it is secondary, that is, it is caused by some other disease like that of the kidneys, treatment of that malady should be started. But if it is of primary origin, a course of treatment to correct the balance of *vata* or *vayu* must be initiated, because all the drugs which alleviate *vayu* are beneficial in this condition.

Lahsuna or garlic is the most important substance helpful in controlling blood pressure. A paste made of about 1 gm of garlic, mixed with a glass of buttermilk, taken twice a day, will help bring the blood pressure to normal. Garlic may be fried in *ghee* if the patient finds the smell offensive, but the medicinal properties of garlic tend to be destroyed with boiling or frying. It should, therefore, be taken raw. Small cloves of garlic (there is a variety which resembles onions) are more helpful than the regular variety. A few cloves of garlic taken raw on an empty stomach in the morning will correct any vitiation of *vata*, whether it is flatulence or blood pressure.

Medicines & Prescriptions: *Sarpagandha* (*Rauwolfia Serpentina*) is another drug which has been used in Ayurveda for many centuries for the treatment of hypertension. Modern medicine has successfully isolated the alkaloids of this drug and it is being used extensively by allopaths. Ayurveda, however, prefers to use the root of the drug in a powdered form. The usual dose is half a teaspoonful of the powder thrice a day. The alkaloids used by the practitioners of modern medicine have some harmful side-effects which are not present in the powder of the root. An overdose of the powder will not have any harmful effects either.

The following prescription is of special significance in the treatment of hypertension: 60 mg of *Rasaraja*, 120 mg of *Pravalapishti Maheshwar*, and 750 mg of *Rasayana* of *Sarpagandha* should be taken thrice daily with *amla* or honey.

Along with this, 1gm of *harada powder*, and 4 gm of *flea seed husk* should be taken at night with water or milk. This will help contain constipation and the bowels will remain clear. If there is dyspepsia along with hypertension, 3 gm of *Yamanishadava* may be given twice after meals with water.

Dhara therapy is also helpful in dealing with obstinate cases of hypertension. Oil boiled with *Bala* (*Side cordifolia*) and milk is allowed to drop in small droplets on the forehead of the patient from a height. The vessel containing it may be suspended from a hook or from the ceiling. The oil drips on the forehead of the patient between the eyes. The same oil may be used for purposes of massage of the patient's body, particularly the head. *Satavartile Kshirabala Taila* may be given internally in five drop doses with a cup of milk.

Diet and Other Regimen: The patient should be kept on a low fat diet; hydrogenated oils and saturated fats must be avoided at all costs. Butter and *ghee* prepared from cow's milk is allowed. Vegetables like bitter gourd and other varieties of gourd and drumsticks should be allowed. The best diet for a patient suffering from hypertension is, of course, boiled vegetables and fruits. Carbohydrates are best avoided as they create digestive complications in such patients.

Complete rest should be advised: the patient must try to sleep early and keep regular habits. Violent exercise should be avoided. A slow walk in the morning is the best exercise for such a patient.

Low Blood Pressure *(Nyuna Raktachap)*

If the pressure of the blood being pumped by the heart into the arteries falls below the average 140 (systolic) and 80 (diastolic), there may be increase in the pulse rate, cold sweats, and a feeling of extreme weakness and giddiness.

Causes and Symptoms: Low blood pressure may be caused by: injury leading to loss of blood, food poisoning, acute or chronic anaemia, and other disorders. If the pressure remains a little lower than the average, it is a healthy sign, because in moments of stress, the heart will be able to deal with any emergency. But if it falls below the minimum necessary for sound health, it should cause worry. The first requirement is to ascertain the cause of the malady. If it is anaemia or sudden loss of blood, these conditions should be treated first. Severe blood loss, as in an injury, may necessitate transfusion of blood. Low blood pressure due to anaemia can be cured only when the persistent lack of blood in the system has been dealt with. For persistent cases of low blood pressure, the medicines mentioned in the section dealing with anaemia should be administered.

Ayurveda maintains that low blood pressure is caused by vitiation of *vayu* and can be treated by drugs which restore the balance of this *dosha* in the body.

Home Remedies: Administration of brandy or alcohol of any variety in quantities from 15 to 50 ml, diluted with warm water, is a temporary expedient which can be tried till the exact cause of the malady is ascertained.

Diet and Other Regimen: A patient suffering from low blood pressure should be given a balanced nutritious diet full of proteins and carbohydrates. Dry fruits; cheese; flesh of chicken, pigeon, rabbit, and goat—in that order; soups of meat and black gram; fruits such as mangoes, bananas, apples, grapes; and leguminous vegetables, such as beans of all varieties, should be the mainstay of the diet of a patient suffering from chronically low blood pressure.

The patient should avoid vigorous exercise and excessive sex. Intoxicants like alcohol and tobacco may be permitted in moderate quantities.

Heart Diseases *(Hridroga)*

The heart is a hollow, muscular pump with four cavities, each provided at its outlet with a valve, whose function is to maintain the circulation of the blood. The heart beats at the rate of 72 per minute in a healthy adult, with the rate of respiration being one-fourth. The blood is pushed out through the arteries, returns through the veins, and is then sent out again. The circulation of the blood in the body is completed in 15 seconds.

Causes and Symptoms: Ancient Ayurvedists recognised the heart as one of the most important organs in the body. The main symptoms produced due to its malfunctioning included generalized weakness, diminished appetite, swelling all over the body, breathlessness, fast respiration, and pulse. It was also known that malfunctioning of different parts of the heart caused other specific symptoms such as constriction in the chest or pain in the chest.

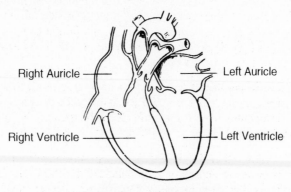

Right Auricle

Left Auricle

Right Ventricle

Left Ventricle

Heart and its Chambers

The detailed working of the heart and the diagnostic procedures for pin-pointing the defective part of the heart are the contribution of modern researchers. The classification of the diseases of the heart into congenital or acquired; those of the endocardium, myocardium, and pericardium; various disorders relating to the conduction of electrical impulses and the production of heart beats, is a modern phenomenon. So also is the fact that the circulation of blood in the coronary arteries nourishes the heart muscle, and its deficiency leads to diseases like angina pectoris, coronary heart disease, and heart attack. Surgical intervention in heart diseases is an entirely modern phenomenon.

According to Ayurveda when *vayu* is vitiated and disturbs the balance of *rasa dhatu* in the body, the various diseases of the heart are born. Ayurveda believes that heart disease may be caused by the vitiation of *vayu, pitta, kapha* or all the three *doshas* taken together, along with certain organisms.

Medicines & Prescriptions: In general cases of heart ailments, the following prescriptions are useful:

1. *Nagarjunabha; Prabhakar Vati; Kukumbhadi Churna.*
   120 mg of *Nagarjunabha*, 240 mg of *Prabhakar Vati*, and 1 gm of *Kukumbhadi Churna* to be taken twice daily with *Pomegranate Syrup.*

2. *Parthadyarishta.*
   24 mg of *Parthadyarishta* to be taken twice with rose water after meals.

3. *Arogyavardhani; Hingugragandhadi Churna.*
   500 mg of *Arogyavardhani* and 2 gm of *Hingugragandhadi Churna* to be taken with water before sleep.

In cases where the heart disease (whatever the technical name) is caused by vitiation of *vayu*, the following drugs are recommended:

1. *Makaradhwaja; Chintamani Rasa; Shringa Bhasma.*
   60 mg of *Makaradhwaja*, 120 mg of *Chintamani Rasa*, and 240 mg of *Shringa Bhasma* to be taken twice, morning and evening.

2. *Pushkaramuladi Churna.*	1 gm of *Pushkaramuladi Churna* to be taken twice after meals with *Vallabhaka Ghrita* or fermented carrots (*kaanji*).
3. *Visheshwara Rasa; Hritpatri Churna* (*digitalis*).	120 mg each of *Visheshwara Rasa* and *Hritpatri Churna* to be taken with sugar candy (*mishri*) last thing at night.

In heart disease caused by vitiation of *pitta*, the following are the drugs of choice:

1. *Panchanana Rasa; Vyomashma Pishti; Drakshadi Churna.*	120 mg each of *Panchanana Rasa* and *Vyomashma Pishti*, and 2 gm of *Drakshadi Churna* to be taken with cold water in the morning and evening.
2. *Arjuna Ghrita.*	12 gm of *Arjuna Ghrita* to be taken once in the morning with *mishri* and cow's milk.

If the heart ailment has been caused by the vitiation of *kapha*, the following should give complete relief:

1. *Hridyarnava Rasa; Shankar Vati; Pipplimula Churna; Powder of seeds of Cardamom.*	120 mg each of *Hridyarnava Rasa* and *Shankar Vati*, and 500 mg each of *Pipplimula Churna* and powder of seeds of cardamom to be taken twice daily.
2. *Arjuna Churna; Krishnadya Churna.*	1 gm of *Arjuna Churna* and 2 gm of *Krishnadya Churna* to be taken with warm water after meals twice daily.

3. *Makaradhwaja;*	60 mg of *Makaradhwaja,*
Prabhakara Vati;	240 mg of *Prabhakara*
Arogyavardhini.	*Vati*, and 50 mg of
	Arogyavardhini to be
	taken with decoction of
	Triphala once before
	sleep.

If heart trouble is due to vitiation of all the three *doshas,* the medicines of choice are:

1. *Ratnakara Rasa;*	120 mg each of
Mukta Pishti;	*Ratnakara Rasa* and
Pushkaramula Churna.	*Mukta Pishti*, and 500
	mg of *Pushkaramula*
	Churna to be taken with
	Arjuna Ghrita in the
	morning and evening.
2. *Chandrodaya;*	60 mg of *Chandrodaya,*
Yakuti;	and 120 mg each of
Digitalis Powder.	*Yakuti* and *Digitalis*
	Powder to be taken twice
	daily.

Diet and Other Regimen: A person suffering from heart disease should eat fat-free foods which can be easily digested. It would be better if the patient can take a salt-free diet. Liquid diets comprising vegetable and meat soups; juices of fruits and even vegetables, such as carrots, should be taken. The best regimen would be a diet of boiled vegetables, free from salt and other condiments.

A strict regimen must be prescribed for a person suffering from any heart ailments. He should never strain his heart; after an attack, he must be given complete bed rest.

The patient should not be disturbed and no worries or strain should mar his daily routine. Exertion of any type should be prohibited. After the attack has passed, he can be allowed to go for walks. Care should be taken that his bowels remain clear so that no flatulence forms in them, as it is likely to depress the diaphragm which, in turn, can give rise to cardiac complaints.

Diseases of the Nervous System

करणायतनेष्वग्र्या बाह्योष्वाभ्यन्तरेषु च ।
निविशन्ते यदा दोषारतदा मूर्च्छन्ति मानवाः ॥

*When a disease attacks on the psychosomatic plane, that is,
when there is both physical and mental morbidity, a person
loses consciousness.*

BHOJARATNAKAR

THE CENTRAL and peripheral nervous system consists of three
parts: the brain and the spinal cord—often spoken of together
as the central nervous system; the nerves which proceed from
the brain and spinal cord—forty-three in number on each side—
named the cerebrospinal or peripheral nerves; the third part
consisting of a number of ganglia-containing nerve cells, which
are profusely connected by plexuses of nerve fibres, and are
situated in the neck, thorax, and abdomen. This part is known
as the autonomic nervous system.

The nerve cells originate or receive impulses and
impressions of various sorts, which are conveyed by them to
the muscles, blood-vessels, and so on, by efferent nerves, or
received by them through afferent nerves coming from the skin,
organs of sense, joints, and other parts of the body. The
autonomic nervous system is concerned mainly with the
movement and other functions of the internal organs, secreting
glands, and blood-vessels, the activities of which proceed
independently of the will. In a sense, the autonomic nervous
system is the controller of all bodily functions.

Nervous diseases are some of the most difficult diseases in so far as their diagnosis and treatment are concerned. The brain and the spinal cord are enclosed in the skull and the spine, beyond the reach of direct examination. Since the nerves everywhere are deeply buried in the tissues, the nature of nervous diseases must be made out from the disturbances of the organs governed by the affected nerves.

Kinds of Disorders

Nervous disorders can broadly be categorised as organic and functional. In the first category are included diseases which result in somatic (body) changes; functional disorders are those where no bodily symptoms can be recognised. Epilepsy, hysteria, and many cases of neuralgia are categorised under functional disorders; whereas, sclerosis, tumours, cysts, ruptures, or blockage in the blood vessels (with consequent loss of nutrition in a part of the brain), and local inflammation constitute an organic change.

Causes and Symptoms: Many factors contribute to the production of nervous diseases. A particular temperament or a peculiar way of life can be one such factor. Some persons, particularly those of great intellectual power and artistic temperament, seem born with a nervous constitution. In this case also, as in the case of some somatic disorders, hereditary factors appear to play an important role. The great pressure of modern life tends to exhaust the nervous system and bring on many diseases. That is why one comes across more cases of nervous disorders among the urban population than among the villagers who are not subjected to the stresses and strains that the city folk are an easy prey to. Shock—both to the mind and the body—such as the loss of a relative, financial reverses, an unfortunate love affair, or an accident may be the starting point of chronic nervous complaints. Many poisons produced within the body during a disease and those taken in from outside, have a specially harmful action upon the nervous system. The chief among them is syphilis, which plays an important role in the production of locomotor ataxia in which there is instability of gait, general paralysis, and certain tumours of the brain and the spinal cord. In advanced life syphilis leads to degenerative changes that bring about premature loss of mental power. Chronic alcoholism may cause severe mental derangement and multiple neuritis.

Many slight afflictions of the nervous system are attributed to defects in the organs controlled by the affected nerves.

There are two main symptoms of nervous diseases: disturbance of sensation, either in the form of loss of feeling, or of great pain, or experiencing perverted sensations such as tingling or hot flushes; else the patient may experience, more or less, complete paralysis of groups of muscles. The nutritional status of all affected organs is impaired in all serious nervous diseases and injuries. As a result, localized sweating, a glassy condition of the skin, bedsores, ulcers, and even gangrene of the limbs are liable to appear in the final stages of nervous maladies. The functions of the internal organs, which are governed by the autonomic system, are not affected unless this system is diseased. The movement of the bowels and bladder are, however, governed by spinal nerves, and thus, these natural functions are impaired in all serious diseases of the spinal cord, so that difficulty of voiding or of retaining the stools and urine is experienced in such cases. When the cranial nerves are involved, definite symptoms arise. Smell, vision, hearing, touch, and all other modalities of sensation are impaired or lost in cases of injury to, or disease of any of the cranial nerves. In some cases, total paralysis may result.

According to Ayurveda, most mental and nervous disorders are due to the vitiation of the three *doshas*: *vata*, *pitta*, and *kapha*. One of the ancient texts opines that persons with a weak will-power and beset with bad habits of eating and drinking fall prey to mental disorders because the three *doshas* are vitiated. Sushruta has advised the physician to enquire into the food and living habits of a patient suffering from nervous or mental disorders before he proceeds to diagnose the malady. Both the somatic and the mental or psychological symptoms have to be studied before a correct diagnosis can be made because, in some cases, the cause may be of bodily weakness. A typical case is that of syncope or fainting. A weak-willed person may not be able to withstand a mental or physical shock

132

and may fall down with syncope. Severe anaemia or cardiac insufficiency caused by the inability of the heart to pump the required amount of blood may also be the cause of the fainting. In some cases, the adrenal gland may be defective and may not be producing the required amount of adrenaline to withstand the mental or physical shock.

Fainting or Syncope *(Murchha)*

Syncope or fainting is a term applied to a temporary loss of consciousness.

Causes and Symptoms: There may be a sudden diminution of blood supply to the brain which may cause fainting. A powerful emotion, like the news of the death of a dear one, and sometimes, great joy, may cause a person to faint. Severe pain due to serious injury in a road accident may result in loss of consciousness. Getting up suddenly from bed after a prolonged period of illness, standing for a long time, disgusting smells and sights—like that of a butcher killing an animal, and general exhaustion are also some of the causes of fainting.

Sushruta has categorised syncope into seven classes depending upon whether it originates from the vitiation of the three *doshas*, blood disorders, alcoholism, or the ingestion of poison into the system. Charaka, however, is of the view that syncope is of four types: three resulting from the vitiation of the various *doshas;* and one—a combination of all the three *doshas*. Fainting may also be due to a vasovagal attack, which results when the venous return of the blood is not maintained.

Medicines & Prescriptions: If the syncope becomes frequent even after removing the somatic causative factors, the following course of treatment is advised:

1. *Murchhantaka Rasa.*	240 mg to be taken in the morning and evening with honey.
2. *Chandravaleha.*	10 gm to be taken with cow's milk at breakfast.

Diet and Other Regimen: A person subject to frequent syncope should avoid intoxicating drinks. Soft, easily-digestible food is recommended.

Morning and evening walks, pleasant surroundings, freedom from worry, and an easy way of life are recommended. Violent exercise is forbidden. Those with a tendency towards introversion should turn to their friends and relatives so that they do not brood over their problems. Such patients should also see that they do not suffer from constipation. A mild purgative may be taken if constipation develops.

Vertigo *(Bhrama)*

Vertigo or giddiness is a condition in which a person loses the power of balancing himself, and experiences a false sensation as to his own movements or those of surrounding objects.

Causes and Symptoms: Some diseases of the ear which may disturb the balance of the fluids in the inner ear may be the causes of giddiness. Some disorders of the stomach; defective eyesight; an impaired functioning of the nervous system, especially of the cerebellum; an attack of migraine; a mild attack of epilepsy; and diseases of the brain, such as a tumour, are some of the other causes. An important cause of vertigo is impaired circulation of the blood in which the vital fluid does not reach the brain in adequate quantities.

Medicines & Prescriptions:

1. *Suvarna Sutashekhara Rasa.*	60 mg to be taken twice daily with decoction of *amla.*
2. *Duralabha Quath.*	50 ml to be taken with 5 ml of *ghee* twice daily.
3. *Saraswatarishta; Ashwagandharishta.*	10 ml each of *Saraswatarishta* and *Ashwagandharishta* to be taken twice daily after meals.

Ashwagandha can be administered in cases of insomnia associated with vertigo.

Diet and Other Regimen: The patient should be kept on an easily-digestible diet and should avoid smoking, drinking, and all narcotic drugs.

He should live in pleasant surroundings and try to keep free from worry. Morning and evening walks, pleasant companionship, and adequate rest are recommended. If there is constipation, 6 gm of *amaltas* should be administered with decoction of *haritiki* at bedtime.

Insomnia *(Anidra)*

Insomnia or sleeplessness is a condition that often causes annoyance, and by depriving the person of his natural rest, results in interference with his activity during the day. When it becomes a habit, it may pose a serious menace to health.

Causes and Symptoms: Insomnia may be due to a variety of causes that keep the person awake altogether, or result in disturbing dreams and unrefreshing slumber. There are many people with a nervous temperament whose sleep is much more liable to be interrupted by trivial causes than that of their easy-going neighbours. In temporary cases of sleeplessness or dreaming in which the affected person suffers from disturbed nights now and then, the cause is usually to be sought in some external source of irritation. A slight degree of pain; uncomfortable surroundings, such as insufficient covering in winter or a hot and humid night without a fan; an overfull stomach causing discomfort; or a nagging worry may prevent the brain from attaining the degree of relaxation which is a prerequisite of sleep. Other factors such as extreme worry overwork, voluntary limitation of the hours of sleep, and grief may lead to a habitual lack of sleep. Poisonous substances circulating in the blood, as in the case of a fever or an infection, neurasthenia, or nervous weakness may also cause loss of sleep.

Medicines & Prescriptions: The treatment of insomnia lies in removing the cause. After the somatic reasons such as dyspepsia, pain, and uncomfortable surroundings have all been removed and sleep still refuses to oblige, the physician must then look for psychological reasons which deny the patient a restful sleep. The vitiation of the three *doshas,* taken together or individually, may be the cause of the disorder. *Brahmi* (*Bacopa monniera*) and *Vacha* (*Acorus calamus*), and, of course, *Amalaki* are the drugs of choice for insomnia. Powders of these drugs, individually or in combination, in doses of one teaspoonful, are given thrice a day with water or milk. *Til* (sesame) oil should be boiled with these powders and used for massaging the head and body before a bath. An alternative remedy is poppy seed oil.

Another remedy which can be administered by a practitioner is *dhara*. Two litres of buffalo milk is boiled with two ounces of *Mustak* (*Cyperus rotundus*) powder and then converted into curd. The curd is then churned and the butter removed. The buttermilk left, mixed with an equal quantity of decoction of *amalaki*, is dropped, one drop at a time, between the eyebrows of the patient when he lies flat on his back. The dripping is continued for fifteen to twenty minutes in the morning. This is followed by a bath. Any of the following standard medicines may also be tried:

1.	*Vatakulantaka.*	120 mg to be administered twice daily with honey.
2.	*Nidrodaya Rasa.*	120 mg to be taken with honey.
3.	*Ashwagandha Churna.*	1 gm to be taken with sugar and *ghee*.
4.	*Pipplimula Churna;*	1.5 gm to be taken in a single dose at bedtime.
	Swarnamakshika.	1 gm to be taken with *gur*.

In addition, *Chameli Taila* should be used for massaging the head to induce sleep.

Home Remedies: A common home remedy for insomnia is the banana. A teaspoonful of fried powder of cumin seeds should be mixed with the pulp of a ripe banana and taken last thing at night. Cow's *ghee* should be used for massaging the soles of the feet at night.

Diet and Other Regimen: The patient should have a filling diet depending on his capacity to digest it. Buffalo milk and its buttermilk are particularly helpful.

136

Massage of the body, followed by a cold or hot bath, depending on the season, are recommended. The patient must take exercise so that he is tired before he lies down in bed. Predisposing causes like worry and mental strain must be removed before one can expect any success in the treatment of insomnia.

Coma *(Sanyas)*

Coma is a state of profound unconsciousness, in which the sufferer cannot be aroused, and there are no reflex movements when the skin is pinched, the eyeball touched, and so on. The breathing is heavy, deep, and akin to snoring, but the heart's function is normal.

Causes and Symptoms: Coma may be caused by high fever, diabetes mellitus, Bright's disease, alcohol, epilepsy, cerebral tumour, meningitis, injury to the head, overdose of insulin, carbon monoxide poisoning, and poisoning with opium and other narcotic drugs. If the condition does not pass off in twenty-four hours, death generally ensues. There have been cases, of course, where coma has continued for months, and, in some cases, for years before death intervened. Here we are dealing with ordinary cases of coma.

According to Ayurveda, vitiation of the three *doshas* depresses the cerebrum so as to produce coma, particularly, in a weak person. An ordinary fit of fainting may subside and the sufferer may feel alright after some time, but coma has to be dealt with by an experienced physician. Some cases of coma may be due to thrombosis, compression, concussion—produced by a blow to the head, cirrhosis of the liver, cerebral malaria, or hypertension.

Medicines & Prescriptions: A comatose person should be revived by strong stimulants. *Kevanch Phali* may be rubbed on his body to revive him. After that, the patient should be laid in a darkened room. If the blood pressure is abnormally high, the patient may be bled; loss of 400 to 500 ml of blood is sure to bring down the pressure. If the coma is due to diabetes mellitus, efforts should be directed towards reducing the amount of sugar present in the blood. The patient should be kept on a restricted diet for a couple of days and be given only liquids while his blood sugar is being monitored.

Any of the following medicines, singly or in combination, may be used to prevent another attack of coma:

1. *Murchhantaka Rasa; Yogendra Rasa; Pravalapishti; Shankhapushpi Churna.*	120 mg each of *Murchhantaka Rasa* and *Yogendra Rasa*, 240 mg of *Pravalapishti*, and 500 mg of *Shankhapushpi Churna* to be taken thrice daily with honey and cow's *ghee*.
2. *Mahakalyanaka Ghrita.*	12 gm to be taken with cow's milk at breakfast.
3. *Ashwagandharishta.*	20 ml to be taken after meals with water, twice daily.
4. *Shri Gopal Taila; Shatavari Taila.*	3 gm of *Shri Gopal Taila* and 6 gm of *Shatavari Taila* should be used for massage of the head and body.

Diet and Other Regimen: An easily-digestible diet is recommended.

Patients are advised to lead a restful life in pleasant surroundings. They should not let constipation develop. Violent exercise, worry, and mental strain are to be avoided. Pleasant companionship, music, and other forms of entertainment have therapeutic value in such cases.

Insanity and Other Mental Disorders

Insanity and other mental disorders are more intractable than somatic or physical diseases. The human brain and its workings are not easy to understand in the best of circumstances, and when the brain is diseased or refuses to function along normal lines, even the best of physicians may be puzzled.

Causes and Symptoms: Mental illness arises from a disease or disordered working of that part of the nervous system which controls the mind and conduct. There are various grades of mental disorders ranging from slight peculiarities to temporary delirium and more.

The causes of mental disorders fall into two groups. Certain persons go through life with a tendency towards becoming disordered mentally when, at any time, certain causes arise. Others may be constantly subjected to much greater strains of the same nature without developing any mental abnormality. It is necessary, therefore, to recognize the nervous constitution of the patient or a set of predisposing causes, and the stresses which are particularly liable to disturb his mind. Among the predisposing causes are: heredity; abnormal disposition or temperament; an over-finely balanced mind subject to going haywire at the slightest provocation; exciting causes which may be in the nature of a sudden shock, exhaustion of the nervous system, infections like those of some fevers, tuberculosis or syphilis, disorders of the endocrine glands, disturbed circulation of blood, alcoholism, and senility or senile degeneration; certain stages in life when the mind may lose its balance, namely, adolescence, childbirth and its complications, the climacteric period around menopause; senile degeneration; and organic diseases of the nervous system.

Mental illness rarely develops suddenly and indications of an approaching mental disorder may be gathered from some early premonitory symptoms, although these may be of so light a character as to escape observation. The most important among them is the alteration of disposition. A person of a suspicious nature may carry his suspicions too far and start looking at everybody as his enemy, bent upon doing him harm. Or the change may be in the opposite direction. The early alterations of habit and conduct are generally accompanied by some physical symptoms such as insomnia, disorders of digestion, and loss of weight.

Regardless of technical names, mental illness falls under two broad categories: insane beliefs and insane acts. The first category includes delusions, perhaps of grandeur or an unseen agency; suspicion and persecution; and hallucinations or false perceptions. The patient may imagine some unknown or unseen persons talking to him and appearing before him in a certain garb. The most serious delusions involve hallucinations of smell. Insane acts may include suicide and homicide, in addition to constant tearing of clothes, fantastic and extravagant dressing or disregard of personal appearance, refusal to eat food, kleptomania or obsessive stealing, dipsomania or obsessive thirst, indecent exposure of the self, and the commission of unnatural sexual offences.

Varieties of Mental Disorders: Mental disorders can be broadly placed in two categories: neuroses and psychoses. The first category is of a mild form in which there is a general emotional tone of anxiety or apprehension: patients are afraid to open letters lest the contents convey bad news, and, by the same reason, they are afraid of telegrams. Persons suffering from a mild indisposition may also interpret the same as a symptom of some fatal disease. Exophthalimic goitre, which is sometimes accompanied by mental symptoms, may be included in this group. Neurasthenia, hysteria and various obsessions including such symptoms as irrepressible thoughts and impulses fall into the group of psychoneuroses.

The other category of mental disorders, namely, psychoses, includes mania, melancholia, manic-depressive psychosis, paranoia, schizophrenia or dementia praecox, and certain confusional states in which there is more of disorientation than any serious disorder. There may be senile dementia and general paralysis of the insane which, in most cases, is the result of syphilis of the nervous system.

Ayurveda recognises a large variety of insanity cases. The causative factors are, of course, vitiation of the three *doshas*, sudden shocks—mental or physical, weakness of the nervous system, ingestion of certain poisons or the formation of certain poisonous substances in the body because of certain diseases.

Medicines & Prescriptions: The old masters have recommended a psychological course of treatment in the earlier stages: for example, the patient who is in a depressed state of mind should be entertained and his mind sought to be diverted from his imaginary problems. If the insanity is of *vatik* origin, that is, if it is because of the vitiation of *vata dosha*, certain preparations of *ghee--Siddha Ghritas*--should be administered. If the insanity is of *pitta* origin, purgatives may be administered and in the case of *kapha* being at the root of the malady, vomiting should be induced. The following medicines are helpful in dealing with most cases of insanity:

1. *Chaturbhuja Rasa; Pravalapishta; Shankhapushpi Churna.*	120 mg of *Chaturbhuja Rasa*, 240 mg of *Pravalapishta*, and 1 gm of *Shankhapushpi Churna* to be taken twice daily with honey.
2. *Rajatabhasma; Chandravaleha.*	80 mg of *Rajatabhasma* and 10 gm of *Chandravaleha* to be given twice daily with cow's milk.
3. *Lashunadya Ghrita.*	12 gm should be mixed with the food of the patient twice daily.
4. *Saraswatarishta.*	20 ml should be taken twice daily with water after meals.

Shatadhauta or Sahasradhauta Ghrita should be used for massaging the head. Castor oil should be administered to the patient twice a week to keep his bowels clear.

Sarpagandha (Rauwolfia serpentina), extensively used in allopathy in the treatment of hypertension, and *Shankhpushpi* should be used in the form of a paste on the forehead. Some of the well-known Ayurvedic preparations to deal with insanity are: *Unmadagajakesari*—240 mg with milk; *Unmadabhanjana Rasa*—240 mg with honey; *Unmadabhanjini Vatika*—to be used as a paste for the eyes; *Bhutankusha Rasa*—240 mg with juice of ginger; *Bhatabhairava Rasa*—240 mg with five seeds of *dhatura* and cow's *ghee;* and *Shivaghrita*—12 mg to 20 mg doses.

Home Remedies: *Bhang (Cannabis indica)* should be ground in goat's milk, and the paste so obtained should be applied to the palms and soles during day and at night.

Diet and Other Regimen: The food should be simple but nutritious.

Patients suffering from mental disorders of all types should be kept away from alcohol and other narcotics. Constipation should be prevented at all costs as that is likely to aggravate the condition. Patients should be handled tactfully and never reminded of their condition. In some cases, when they complain of persecution, they may have to be humoured before an effort is made to dispel their misconceptions. A pleasant, understanding atmosphere and companionship are of vital importance in bringing about a cure.

Epilepsy *(Apasmara)*

Epilepsy or falling sickness is a term applied to a nervous disorder characterised by a fit of sudden loss of consciousness, and attended with convulsions.

Causes and Symptoms: In most cases, an attack of epilepsy comes on suddenly, but in some cases, there are premonitory symptoms like a change in the disposition of the patient. There may be an unusual elevation or depression of spirits. Some peculiar symptoms immediately precede the attack: the patient may experience a strong smell; there may be tremors or contractions in a part of the body, and even some extraordinary visions. These premonitory symptoms sometimes give the patient sufficient time to lie down before the fit comes on, and he can avoid the injury which would be sustained if he suddenly fell unconscious.

The seizures are generally preceded by a loud cry: this is not due to any sense of fright or pain, but due to a mere involuntary contraction of the muscles of the larynx and the expulsion of air through the narrowed glottis. If the patient is standing, he suddenly falls and sustains an injury, which may be serious in some cases. He lapses into total unconsciousness; his muscles contract; his head turns towards one side; and his breathing is temporarily arrested. The countenance is more pale than livid, the pupils dilated, and the pulse rapid. This is the first stage of the fit and lasts for about half a minute, and then there is contraction of the muscles and the whole body is thrown into violent agitation. The eyes roll wildly, the teeth are gnashed together, and the tongue is often severely bitten. The breathing is noisy, and foam, flecked with blood, spouts from the sides of the mouth. This stage may last from a few seconds to some minutes, and then the convulsion subsides, the muscles relax, and there is a partial return of consciousness. This is followed by drowsiness and stupor which may continue for some hours, after which the patient wakes up, either completely recovered, or fatigued and depressed.

An epileptic fit may be succeeded by others, one after the other, for long periods. If the patient is subject to fits during the night, it may take longer to recognise the condition and he may wake up in the morning with a peculiar sense of loss. In some cases, however, the fit may come in the form of a total loss of consciousness without any convulsive spasms. In other cases of a more serious nature, the attack may be followed by violent acts on the part of the patient which render him more dangerous. After an attack of epilepsy, the patient may perform acts which he is totally unaware of after his recovery.

According to modern medicine, an epileptic fit occurs when the brain suddenly discharges electrical energy which is devoid of any purposive action, and which takes place from time to time in an unusual manner. The disease may appear at any age, but, more often, the fits start before adult life—usually during infancy or at puberty. Sudden fright, prolonged anxiety, overwork, and alcoholism may bring on the disease in predisposed persons. Ayurveda, however, believes that the disease is due to the vitiation of any of the three *doshas* or all of them. It categorises epilepsy into four types, depending upon the vitiation of a particular *dosha*.

Medicines and Prescriptions: The main objective of treatment of this condition is to strengthen the heart and the nervous system.

Brahmi (*Bocopa monniera*) and *Vacha* (*Acorus calamus*) are the two drugs which are of particular use in this condition. One teaspoonful of *Brahmi* juice or the powder of the root of *Vacha*, or both of them together, should be mixed with honey and given thrice daily. A compound preparation *Brihat Vata Kulantaka Rasa*, which contains the calx of gold, is recommended in two grain doses thrice daily.

143

The following prescriptions are recommended in intractable cases of epilepsy:

1. *Jatamansi Churna; Smritisagara Rasa; Vacha Churna.*
   1 gm of *Jatamansi Churna*, 120 mg of *Smritisagara Rasa*, and 1 gm of *Vacha Churna* to be taken twice daily with honey.

2. *Mahakalyanaka Ghrita.*
   10 gm to be taken twice daily with candied sugar and cow's milk.

3. *Saraswatarishta.*
   20 ml to be taken twice daily after meals with water.

4. *Apasmarantaka Rasa.*
   120 mg to be taken twice daily with honey.

Along with this, 50 ml of the urine of the female ass may be given twice daily to the patient. Sesame oil should be used for the massage of the head and the soles of the feet.

Diet and Other Regimen: The diet of the epilepsy patient should consist mainly of milk. Easily-digested foods, fruits and vegetables—mostly green, should form the rest of the diet.

A daily cold bath, light exercise, and a clean life are helpful. Mental strain should be avoided.

Hysteria *(Yoshapasmara)*

Hysteria is a neurosis which manifests itself by overaction of some parts of the nervous system.

Causes and Symptoms: The symptoms of hysteria are convulsive seizures, spasms and contractions of the limbs, paralysis, loss of sensation over areas of the body, and affliction of the various internal organs. Most of these symptoms are the result of auto-suggestion and are readily relieved by suggestion from another person.

Ayurveda regards hysteria as another form of epilepsy. The condition is far more common among women than in men. Faulty upbringing during childhood predisposes a person to hysteria. Young women with somewhat unequally developed minds and pampered habits can become hysterical due to sudden fright, family worries, grief, or a love affair. Mental changes occur among victims of hysteria. They become whimsical, are dominated by certain fixed ideas, and prove incapable of the same work and concentration as before. They become more excitable and hypersensitive.

Convulsive hysteria is the most marked form of hysteria. An attack provoked by some excitement may begin with laughter or weeping, or may give no warning sign. The victim falls into a semi-conscious or unconscious condition. The difference between an epileptic fit and a hysterical fit is that the victim of epilepsy falls down suddenly, injuring himself, whereas a hysterical patient gently subsides into a chair or on to the floor. She moans, moves her head from side to side, and rolls her eyes. During this stage, she may see visions and exhibit powerful emotions of fear, ecstasy, or joy. Loss of sensation in some parts of the body is often noticed. In some cases, it may even resemble paralysis. The other manifestations are spasms and contractions of the muscles, leading to some deformity if the muscles are too tightly pulled during a fit.

The paralysis accompanying hysteria is generally of a psychological origin, passing off if the attention is strongly diverted or somebody is able to mentally affect the patient. In some cases, the muscles of the larynx become paralyzed and the victim may go about like a mute person for years before some powerful influence forces her to exert her will and the voice box becomes active again.

Hysteria affects only those people who have a weak will-power and are given to fantasies of suffering. In some cases there may be some changes that take place in the internal organs of the body. Constant hiccups, barking noises, excessive vomiting, diarrhoea, absolute loss of appetite, and profound changes in blood circulation may take place. A joint, especially of the hip or the knee, may become swollen, stiff, and painful and may remain so for months.

Medicines and Prescriptions: Hysteria can be treated by following the same regimen of medication as has been indicated for epilepsy.

Diet and Other Regimen: The patient can continue to take a normal diet.

Hysterical patients should be tactfully but firmly handled. They should not be allowed to while away their time in useless pursuits. Enough work to occupy them should be provided, and most important of all, they should not be pampered. They should be exhorted to strengthen their power of resistance and told that there is nothing wrong with them. Techniques of suggestion should be applied to bring them to full recovery. Persuasion, psychoanalysis, education, and employment are important in the treatment of hysteria.

Loss of Memory *(Smutibhransh)*

Memory entails retention of the knowledge of an event and the power to recall. There are some 600 million nerve cells in the brain united together with numberless fibres into countless combinations which constitute what we call our memory. The fibres connecting the cells are known as association fibres; they provide the link between two objects and their knowledge. Sound memory depends on the rational grouping of ideas of things in the mind, so that one may call upon the other. The man who ponders most over the occurrences of his daily life will, other things being equal, have the best memory. But no training will make up for a deficiency of nerve cells and association fibres, which are inborn characteristics.

Causes and Symptoms: Memory may be impaired by concussion of the brain or by certain diseases. Old age or senile degeneration of the brain and its cells may lead to loss of memory. Temporary loss of memory, in which the patient forgets even his own identity, may be the result of an injury. These instances are, however, multiplied in film and fiction more than in reality.

Medicines & Prescriptions: Ayurveda has remedies which can improve the power of retention and recall of events, which are, in essence, what we know as the capacity for memory. The drug *Brahmi* is popularly used for improvement of memory. Both its varieties, *Matsyaksi (Bacopa monnieri)* and *Mandukaparni (Centella asiatica)*, are equally useful in promoting memory. An ounce of the juice of the plants is given to the patient on an empty stomach twice daily. *Brahmi* is boiled in cow's *ghee* and the *ghee* attains the qualities inherent in the drug. A teaspoonful of the *ghee* is given twice daily to the patient on an empty stomach; if he is emaciated, the medicine is given with a glass of warm milk and sugar.

Another remedy commonly used in cases of weak memory is the root of *Vacha*. One teaspoonful of the powdered root of the plant is given twice daily with honey and cow's milk. Almond oil and preserve of *amla* are also useful.

Diet and Other Regimen: A nourishing diet with lots of fruits and vegetables should be taken.

The patient should remain free of worry and live amidst pleasant surroundings and companionship. According to yogic procedures, meditation for some time also helps in improving the memory.

Paralytic Afflictions *(Pakshaghat)*

In this section, we shall deal with paralysis in its various forms, partial or total, that afflict grown-ups or children.

Paralysis or palsy means loss of muscular power due to interference with the nervous system. When muscular power is weakened as the result of some affection of the nervous system, the term applied is paralysis. Various technical names are given to various forms of the disease. **Hemiplegia** is applied to paralysis affecting one part of the face, along with the corresponding arm and leg. **Diplegia** means a condition of more or less total paralysis. **Monoplegia** is the paralysis of a single limb; and **paraplegia** signifies paralysis of both sides of the body below a given level, usually from about the level of the waist. **Creeping paralysis** is a vague term applied most often to locomotor ataxia; **shaking paralysis** is the popular name for *paralysis agitans;* and **wasting paralysis** commonly means progressive muscular atrophy.

Causes and Symptoms: Paralysis is classified according to whether it depends on the disease of the brain, spinal cord, or nerves: hence the terms--cerebral, spinal, and peripheral paralysis. The most common form of paralysis due to brain disease is hemiplegia which arises from a disease of the hemisphere of the brain opposite to the side of the body affected. It may occur due to haemorrhage in the brain or blocking of the blood-vessels. One side of the body loses all muscular tone and the muscles hang loose. Trembling palsy, also called *paralysis agitans*, Parkinsonism, or shaking paralysis is characterised by rhythmical tremors and rigidity of the muscles. It is a chronic disease of advanced life and is due to degenerative changes in the base of the cerebrum. At first, symptoms appear in the form of involuntary trembling of the limbs which ceases during sleep. Cerebral palsy is characterised by varying degrees of paralysis, generally, spastic paralysis. Paraplegia is the paralysis of both lower extremities, including usually the lower portion of the trunk. It is sometimes the result of injuries to the spinal column. Wasting palsy is a disease of middle age. It is characterised by the gradual wasting of certain muscles or groups of muscles, loss of power in them, twitching of the muscle fibres, and alteration of tendon and skin reflexes. Progressive muscular atrophy results from these symptoms and is caused by a process of degeneration in the motor cells in the cerebral cortex, the cells of grey matter of the spinal cord, and the nerve cells in the brain. Facial paralysis is another variety of the disease which attacks the muscles of the face.

Medicines & Prescriptions: The following prescriptions, either singly or in combination with others, may be tried:

1. *Rasnadi Quath.*	50 ml to be taken daily.
2. *Ashwagandha Churna; Chopcheeni Churna; Vatavidhwamsana Rasa; Pippali Mula.*	1 gm each of *Ashwagandha Churna* and *Chopcheeni Churna*; 60 mg of *Vatavidhwamsana Rasa* and 1 gm of *Pippali Churna* to be taken thrice daily.
3. *Medicated Castor oil.*	20 ml to be given in the morning with milk.

4. *Mashabaladi Quath;* *Asafoetida;* *Rock salt.*	50 ml *Mashabaladi Quath*, 60 mg *Asafoetida*, and 500 mg *Rock salt* to be used as nasal drops opposite to the side affected.
5. *Brihat Vatachintamani Rasa;* *Ashwagandha Churna.*	30 mg *Brihat Vatachintamani Rasa* and 1 gm *Ashwagandha Churna* to be taken twice daily with meat soup.
6. *Mahanarayana Taila.*	20 ml to follow No 5 above; it should be mixed with milk.
7. *Rasaraja.*	120 mg to be taken last thing at night with milk.

In addition, *Kupiloo Taila* should be rubbed on the affected part. *Siddha Makaradhwaja*, *Malla Chandrodaya*, *Trailokya Chintamani*, *Vatanashan Rasa*, *Navagrahi Shiroraja* are some of the other standard Ayurvedic preparations helpful in dealing with paralysis. If needed, they may be combined with any of the above seven prescriptions.

Diet and Other Regimen: Light, easily-digestible food should be taken.

The patient is advised to undergo physiotherapy for the afflicted parts of his body so as to sustain their strength.

Poliomyelitis
(Shaishaviya Angaghata or Balapakshaghata)

Poliomyelitis, commonly referred to as polio, is a form of infantile paralysis which mostly attacks children.

Causes and Symptoms: Allopathy believes that poliomyelitis is the result of an infectious disease involving the spinal cord and the brain. It starts as a slight indisposition in the child when he may be a little 'off colour'. Fever is followed by loss of muscle tone, and finally, paralysis. In some cases, paralysis of the limbs may come on quite suddenly, usually with a sharp rise in temperature. The child may go to bed in seemingly good health, but may wake up totally paralysed the next morning. The severity of the disease depends on which internal organ has been seriously affected. If the respiratory muscles have been affected, it may bring on death, but if only the spinal cord is affected, and most often that is the case, the lower limbs may be paralysed. If untreated, the leg muscles may atrophy, giving the limbs a dried-up look. Modern medicine has developed a vaccine, available in the form of drops, which gives immunity to infants against polio.

Ayurveda maintains that the various forms of paralysis known as *Pakshaghata*, *Ardhangaghata*, *Ekangaghata* and *Sarvangaghata* are the result of the vitiation of *vata*.

Medicines and Prescriptions: In the initial stages of polio, that is, the first three weeks, the following line of treatment can be adopted with advantage:

1. *Balachaturbhadra Churna; Mukta Pishti.* — 1 gm *Balachaturbhadra Churna* and 30 gm *Mukta Pishti* to be taken thrice daily with powdered cardamom and honey.

2. *Medicated Castor oil.* — 5 ml to be given early morning with *Rasnadi* and *Dashamoola Quath.*

3. *Dhara Sweda.* — Pouring of warm decoctions over the affected organs from a height of four inches is recommended. The decoctions should be made of the drug mentioned in No. 2 above.

After three weeks, the following line of treatment should be adopted:

1. *Rajat Bhasma; Yasad Bhasma; Seesaka Bhasma.* — 15-30 mg of *Rajat Bhasma*, 30-60 mg of *Yasad Bhasma*, 15-30 mg of *Seesaka Bhasma* to be taken twice daily with decoction of *Prasarini (Paedaria foctida).*

2. *Mahanarayana Taila.* This should be used for massaging the affected parts. Fomentation is recommended with a pounded mass of garlic, rock salt, *ajwain*, horse gram, cotton seed, black gram, castor seeds, linseed– tied in a piece of cloth.

A hot water bag may be used to relieve pain.

Diet and Other Regimen: The patient is advised to take light, easily-digestible food.

Physiotherapy is recommended for the afflicted parts of the body. In case of constipation, a glycerine enema should be given.

Cramps *(Khalani)*

Cramps are painful spasmodic contractions of the muscles, occurring most frequently in the limbs, but also apt to affect certain internal organs. This disorder belongs to the class of diseases known as local spasms, of which other varieties exist in such afflictions as spasmodic asthma, tetany, and colic.

Causes and Symptoms: The cause of cramps resides in the nervous system and troubles come on suddenly—sometimes during sleep, when one finds one's leg or arm muscles cramped and bunched together, resulting in acute pain.

The trouble is of a temporary nature and leaves the sufferer as suddenly as it had come. Here we shall deal with one variety which has a tendency to become permanent and that is known as **writer's cramp.** This disorder owes its name to the relative frequency with which it develops in persons who are in the habit of writing too much, although it is by no means confined to them.

The symptoms are, in the first instance, a gradually increasing difficulty experienced in conducting the movements required for writing. The muscles of the fingers and the forearms are seized with cramps. Sometimes the fingers, instead of being cramped, move in a disordered fashion and the pen cannot be grasped, and at other times, the fingers are struck with paralysis and they are unable to move enough to write. It is notable that the movements needed for other functions can be made by the fingers.

Medicines & Prescriptions: The following course of treatment is indicated for writer's cramp:

1. *Bala Quath.*	25 ml to be used as nasal drops thrice daily.
2. *Chandraprabha Vati.*	500 mg to be taken twice daily.
3. *Ashwagandharishta.*	24 ml to be taken twice daily with water after No. 2 above.

The affected hand should be massaged with *Kupiloo oil*. Hot fomentation with a bag of salt should be applied.

Diet and Other Regimen: Milk and its preparations should be taken to increase the intake of calcium.

The patient should be advised to rest his hand for a few weeks.

Sciatica *(Gridhrasi)*

Sciatica is one of the most common forms of neuralgia or pain in the nerves. It affects the great sciatic nerve which emerges from the pelvis and runs down the back of the thigh.

Causes and Symptoms: Sciatica is, in many instances, traceable to exposure to cold and damp. Any pressure on the nerve within the pelvis, such as may be produced by a tumour, may excite an attack of sciatica. Pressure upon a nerve by a prolapsed intervertebral disc between the fourth and the fifth lumber vertebrae is not an uncommon cause of pain along the course of the sciatic nerve. The pain which is felt a little behind the hip joint at first, steadily increases in severity and extends along the course of the nerve and its branches, as far as the toes. The painful points are where the nerve emerges from the pelvis at the lower margin of the buttocks, and around the knee and ankle joints.

Ayurveda believes that sciatica is caused by the aggravation of *vayu*. Sometimes the vitiation of *kapha* along with *vata* brings on the attack. At times constipation precipitates or aggravates an attack of sciatica.

Medicines & Prescriptions: *Eranda* (*Ricinus comumunis*) is the drug of choice for sciatica. A linctus, *Eranda paka*, is given in doses of two teaspoonfuls at bedtime with a cup of warm water or milk. It helps patients with costiveness because *Eranda* or castor acts as a laxative. *Yogaraja Guggulu* is another medicine which is administered in doses of two tablets, four times a day, with water or milk. *Saindhavadi Taila* or *Mahavishagarbha Taila* is recommended for massaging the affected parts, after which hot fomentation should be applied. The limb should be covered with a warm cloth to maintain the heat. *Guggulu Tiktaka Ghrita*—50 ml, and honey—10 ml, may be given as a retention enema. Hot fomentation with a bag of salt is useful in ameliorating the pain of sciatica. The following prescriptions are also recommended:

1. *Vataganjakusha; Vaishwanara Churna.*	240 mg of *Vataganjakusha* and 3 gm of *Vaishwanara Churna* to be taken twice daily after meals with warm water or decoction of *Manjishta.*
2. *Castor oil.*	20 ml should be taken just before sleeping at night with urine of cow.

Diet and Other Regimen: Pulses, beans, and fried foods should be prohibited. Curds and other sour substances should be avoided. Saffron, in small quantities, should be mixed with milk and given to the patient to drink.

Gentle exercise of the leg is advised. Exposure to damp and cold should be avoided. Swimming in warm water is a good exercise for legs.

The patient should use a hard bed and wear a lumbo-sacral belt. Yogic exercises like *Halasana*, *Shalabhasana*, and *Bhujangasana* may be undertaken after pain has subsided to prevent recurrence of sciatica.

Diseases of the Digestive System

आयुर्वर्णो बलं स्वास्थ्यमत्साहोपचयौ प्रभा ।
ओजस्तेजोऽग्रय: प्राणाश्रोक्ता देहाग्निहेतुका: ॥
शान्तेऽग्रौम्रियते, युक्ते चिरं जीवत्यनामय: ।
रोगी स्याद्विकृते, मूलमग्निरतरमान्निरुच्यते ॥

The lifespan, complexion, vitality, good health, zest, plumpness, glow, vital essence, lustre, heat, and life breath are maintained because of agni. When agni (thermogenetic process) is extinguished, man dies; a man endowed with it adequately lives a long and healthy life. When its balance is vitiated, he begins to ail. Therefore the thermal function is said to be the mainstay of life.

CHARAKA SAMHITA

BEFORE STUDYING digestive disorders, we should understand the process of digestion; only then can we properly understand the disorders and their treatment.

The Process of Digestion

The stomach is one of the vital organs of the body, being one of the five so categorised; the other four are the heart, lungs, kidneys, and the brain. The stomach not only stores food during the process of digestion, but also makes it more permeable through the juices it produces. The stomach has minute glands from which gastric juice is produced. The gastric juice helps to break down the food into smaller molecules. The acid in the stomach aids the action of the digestive enzymes. The moment food enters the stomach, the acid starts a churning action to mix the food with the gastric juice so that it becomes absorbable. Light foods like milk and fatless cereals or fruits

154

take much less time to be digested than heavy foods like fried substances which contain fat.

The partially digested food from the stomach enters the intestine and is exposed to the action of bile, pancreatic juice, intestinal juice, and bacteria. The food is, thus, broken down into various absorbable substances which are vital for the growth and development of the body. It is only when the food has passed out from the intestine that the process of digestion is completed and the process of absorption starts. That is how the human body replaces the energy that has been expended.

Ancient Ayurvedists have recognised thirteen types of *agnis*, of which the most important is the *jatharagni*, the others being the seven *dhatu agnis* and five *bhuta agnis*. The *jatharagni*, contained in the *pachaka pitta*, is the root of all the *agnis* of the body. The diminution of *jatharagni* gives rise to most disorders of the stomach, particularly anorexia and dyspepsia. In addition to this *agni* which is the sheet anchor of digestion,

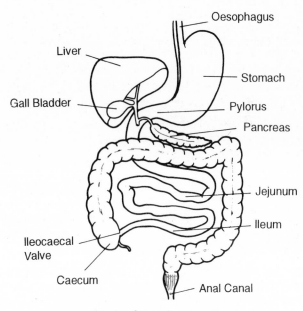

Gastro-intestinal tract

there are six factors which help digestion: *pachaka pitta, samana vayu,* moisture, *kledaka kapha,* time, and a proper combination of the first five. *Vayu* propels the food into the stomach, bringing it near the *agni,* and also inflames the *agni;* moisture breaks up the compactness of the food; *kapha* softens the food. Time is required for completing the process of digestion, and a proper combination of all factors is vital for completing the process of digestion.

We shall now deal with the common disorders of the digestive system in the order of their frequency.

Constipation *(Koshtabadhata)*

The most common disorder is, perhaps, constipation. Those leading an easy, sedate life in a city and consuming rich food are more prone to it than others.

Causes and Symptoms: The main symptom of this disorder is the urge to void the stools but the inability to do so. If constipation continues for some time, it may lead to a feeling of heaviness in the abdomen, and later, headaches, lethargy, loss of appetite, and total apathy. The inability of the intestines to expel the waste matter leads to putrefaction and flatulence. Constipation continuing over a long period may lead to distension of the stomach and severe discomfort.

Home Remedies: In the absence of any organic obstruction, change of food habits is, perhaps, the ideal way to deal with constipation rather than the use of drugs of any kind. If the disorder is due to the habit of taking excessively spiced, fatty foods and highly refined cereals, the first step in dealing with constipation is to advise the patient to take light foods like milk, fruit juices, and boiled vegetables, and totally abstain from fats and refined foods. The patient should be advised to take sufficient amount of liquids—water, milk, and so on—which reduce the dryness of the intestines.

Medicines & Prescriptions: In the case of children suffering from obstinate constipation, a suppository made of macerated leaves of *harita manjari* (*Acalypha indica*) should be introduced into the rectum. An alternative is a suppository

156

made of the stalk of betel leaf and coated with castor oil. Or a poultice made of the leaves of *kidamari* (*Aritolochia bracteata*) should be applied over the abdomen of the child.

The other remedies which tend to relieve constipation are: Powder of *madhuka* (liquorice root) taken with *gur* and water; decoction of *akashbel* (dodder); the pulp of the roots of *arni* (*Clerodendrum phlomidia*) taken with *ghee*; *Isabgol* (flea seed)—two heaped tablespoons—taken with milk or water; castor oil seeds in small doses; Senna, one part, and *harada*, half a part, finely powdered taken in one gram doses thrice daily. Any one or a combination of the above may be tried.

In cases of chronic constipation, pills made with the following ingredients may be tried:

Rose buds	5 parts
Senna leaves	4 parts
Pulp of amaltas	3 parts
Harad	5 parts

Alternatively:

Nishottar	2 parts
Pippali	4 parts
Harada	5 parts
Gur	(equal to the quantity of the substances enumerated above)

If the constipation is associated with dry, hard, and lumpy stools, *jhohar* (*Euphorbia nerifolia*) should be cooked as a pot herb and eaten before meals. *Harada* should be fried in *ghee* or castor oil and the powder made out of it should be taken with black salt.

Standard medicines available in the market are: *Swadishta Virechan, Lasuna Kshira,* and *Avipittakar Churna.*

Diet and Other Regimen: A patient suffering from chronic constipation should be advised to avoid starchy foods and take leafy vegetables like spinach, cabbage, *chulai,* stalk of mustard (*sarson ka saag*); and fruits like musk melon, papaya, and mangoes.

The patient should also take long walks and light exercise which will tone up his stomach muscles. A glass of water taken in the morning also helps in proper bowel habits.

Dyspepsia *(Agnimandya)*

Dyspepsia or indigestion is the term applied to difficulty in digesting food.

Causes and Symptoms: Dyspepsia may be associated with pain in the region of the stomach, flatulence, eructations, a foul taste in the mouth, heartburn, and a general feeling of discomfort. There is also loss of appetite in some cases of dyspepsia. Irregular food habits in the form of overeating or eating at the wrong time, or the wrong type of food leads to indigestion.

The general term applied to the symptoms associated with dyspepsia in Ayurveda is *Agnimandya,* which is a decreased digesting capacity of *agnis*, particularly, *jatharagni*, which aids digestion. The aggravation of the *doshas—vata, pitta,* and *kapha*—leads to this disease. Excess of *vata* leads to pain in the stomach; that of *pitta* causes a burning sensation; and if *kapha* is vitiated, there is nausea and vomiting.

Home Remedies: As in constipation, it is easier to prevent dyspepsia than to cure it, if one follows the simple rules enunciated by Ayurveda. Fresh and hot food should be taken in pleasant surroundings. It should be taken only when the previous meal has been properly digested. Foods which do not agree with each other should be avoided. One should never eat in a hurry or when worried or angry. Emotions like anger and worry, and tensions of modern life, will inevitably lead to dyspepsia. One should avoid eating if heaviness is present. The quantity of food taken should be enough to assuage one's hunger without producing a sense of fullness.

The quantity of food to be ingested varies from individual to individual. A cardinal rule to follow in the matter of food is to avoid *excess*. Some people turn into gluttons, whereas others, though their number is limited, subsist on very little food. Sleep and food are really matters of habit; they can be increased or decreased within certain limits without, in any way, impairing one's health. The human body is a wonderful machine; it adjusts itself to circumstances very quickly, much more quickly than the human mind does. Excess food not only puts too much of load on the digestive system, it is also thrown out of the body in an undigested or incompletely digested form. The quantity of food needed to nourish the body also varies according to the seasons. In summer you need more intake of liquids than of solid foods, whereas in winter it is the reverse. In winter unctuous, sour, and saline foods, flesh of birds and aquatic animals, wines and strong alcoholic beverages may be taken without any harm; but in summer, cooling drinks, milk, rice, and flesh of animals dwelling in forests are the proper foods. Wines should be avoided in summer, except when they are diluted with water.

For chronic indigestion, chew about 1 gm of ginger with powder of rock salt before meals.

Medicines & Prescriptions: An Ayurvedic preparation marketed for dyspepsia is *Hingvashtaka Churna*, the major ingredients of which are *hing* (*asafoetida*), *shunthi* (*Zingiber officinale*), *pippali* (*Piper longum*), *maricha* (*Piper nigrum*), *ajamoda* (*Carum roxburghianum*), *jiraka* (*Cuminum cyminum*), and black cumin seed. The remedy acts best when taken with buttermilk after food. Or it may be taken with the first morsel of food. One teaspoon of the preparation may also be mixed with an equal quantity of *ghee* and taken twice daily. In cases of pain accompanying dyspepsia, another medicine is *Mahashanka Vati*, two tablets of which should be taken thrice daily with warm water. Other prescriptions of choice are:

1. *Ajirnadi Rasa;* *Shatapatriyadi Churna.*	3/4 gm of *Ajirnadi Rasa* and 2 gm of *Shatapatriyadi Churna* to be taken in the morning and evening with warm water.
2. *Draksharishta.*	20 ml to be taken with water twice daily, after meals.
3. *Haritaki Churna;* *Raisins;* *Sugar.*	3 gms each of *Haritaki Churna* and raisins; and 6 gm of sugar to be taken at night with water.

4. *Agnimukha Lavana;* *Narayan Churna.*	1 gm each of *Agnimukha Lavana* and *Narayan Churna* to be taken thrice daily with warm water.
5. *Lashunadi Vati;* *Samudradi Churna;* *Sarjikasatva.*	1 gm each of *Lashunadi* *Vati, Samudradi Churna,* and *Sarjikasatva* to be taken twice daily with warm water after meals.

Diet and Other Regimen: Easily-digestible food with very little or no spices should be taken. Fried foods should be avoided. Light exercise, preferably, morning walks are recommended.

Diarrhoea *(Atisar)*

Diarrhoea, or loose and frequent evacuation of the bowels, is a serious condition. It can be broadly categorised into two types: ordinary diarrhoea and infantile diarrhoea.

Ordinary Diarrhoea

Ordinary diarrhoea occurs frequently and has numerous causes.

Causes and Symptoms: Diarrhoea may occur due to the incapacity of the bowels to cope with heavy fatty foods; ingestion of poisonous substances; certain harmful bacteria, as in cholera or typhoid fever; intake of improper diet; ulceration of the intestines as in tuberculosis or some diseases of the liver, kidneys, lungs, or the heart. Diarrhoea may also be caused by sudden fright or shock due to the death of a beloved one, or worrying too much. The moment the causative worry or shock wears off, it stops automatically without the need for any drugs. But in other cases, a wise physician tries to ascertain the cause and treat it accordingly. Other causes of diarrhoea include: change of climate, as with mountaineers when they reach heights; change of season, as in spring or autumn; and change of diet to which a person is habituated.

Ayurveda recognises many varieties of diarrhoea, but emphasizes mainly on six varieties: those caused by *vata, pitta,* and *kapha;* diarrohea caused by a combination of all the three

160

doshas; diarrhoea caused by sudden fright; *aamaja atisar* caused by indigestion or *amadosha,* which Charaka has categorised as arising from sudden fright. It should be mentioned that Sushruta has classified the diarrohea caused by fright as the one caused by *vata dosha.*

Home Remedies: In diarrhoea of ordinary intensity, preparations made of the various parts of the *babul tree (Gum acacia)* are useful. A mixture of equal parts of the tender leaves of the tree with white *zeera* (cumin seeds) and black *zeera* (caraway seeds) should be administered in doses of 12 gm each, thrice daily. An infusion made of the bark of the tree, comprising about a couple of ounces boiled in a *pint* of water, should be given thrice daily. Another useful remedy is to soak 3 gms of *catechu,* and 4 gm *cinnamon* for two hours in half a *pint* of boiling water, and to give the decoction in 10 ml doses, thrice a day. A powder of dried fruits of *jambul* (rose apple) and decorticated mango seeds can be given in doses of 750 mg to 2 gm thrice daily. Tender aerial roots of the banyan tree macerated in rice water should be given with buttermilk. Alternatively, powder of shelled seed of mango can be given in doses of 1 to 2 gm.

Before mentioning well-known Ayurvedic preparations, let us mention other remedies which are of use in checking diarrhoea. Decoction of the rind and the bark of the pomegranate tree, the paste of the roots of the tamarind tree, the powder of the flowers of the *dhataki* tree (*Woodfordia fruitcosa*), flea seeds or their husk, decoction of the roots of Kurchi (*conessi*), and the root bark of *tarwar* (*tanner's cassia*) and powder of long pepper (*pippali*) are of use.

Medicines & Prescriptions: There are well-known Ayurvedic prescriptions prescribed by the *vaid* in cases of diarrhoea. Any one of them can be tried at a time.

1. *Kutaja Churna; Gangadhara Churna; Hingavashtaka Churna.* — 1 gm each of *Kutaja Churna, Gangadhara Churna* and *Hingavashtaka Churna* to be taken with likewarm water or buttermilk.

2. *Raman Churna; Mahagandhaka Yoga; Sanjivani.*	240 mg each of *Raman Churna* and *Mahagandhaka Yoga;* and 120 mg of *Sanjivani* to be taken thrice with dried cumin seeds, aniseeds and honey.
3. *Shankha Bhasma; Shunthyadi Churna; Bhaskara Lavana.*	120 mg of *Shankha Bhasma,* with 1 gm each of *Shunthyadi Churna* and *Bhaskara Lavana* to be taken thrice daily with water after meals.
4. *Piyushvalli Rasa; Kutaja Churna.*	240 mg of *Piyushvalli Rasa* and 500 mg of *Kutaja Churna* to be taken thrice daily with fleaseed husk.
5. *Rasanjanadi Churna; Yamani Shadava.*	15 gm of *Rasanjanadi Churna* and 1.5 gm of *Yamani Shadava* to be taken twice daily after meals.

Diet and Other Regimen: A liquid or semi-liquid diet should be taken, soups of various vegetables being indicated. Fluid loss should be compensated by intake of oral fluids.

Infantile Diarrhoea

Infantile diarrhoea falls into a separate category and we shall deal with it first. Contaminated milk or infection in the alimentary canal may cause diarrhoea in infants, and if an infant is breast fed, some of the digestive disorders of the mother may be transmitted to the child. Infantile diarrhoea may be accompanied by vomiting or griping pain in the stomach. It is a common disorder at the time of teething. The child refuses milk, is given to crying, and cannot sleep. Care should be taken in such a condition as continued diarrhoea may lead to dehydration.

Medicines & Prescriptions: The 'gripe water' generally marketed for infants contains carminatives which are harmful if administered for a long time. Ayurvedic treatment for infantile diarrhoea consists of administering 150 mg of a paste made out of the root of the *musta* (*Cyperus rotundus*) plant, three to four times a day. If taken in powdered form, 75 mg of the substance, mixed with a teaspoonful of honey, should be given three to four times a day. In case the stools are watery and there is vomiting, 75 mg of the powder of the seed of *jaiphal* (nutmeg) should be given. The essential oil in the nutmeg relieves the griping pain of the infant instantly.

An Ayurvedic preparation marketed as *Gorochanadi Vatika* is of particular use in this condition. A 25 mg pill of this medicine is recommended four times a day till diarrhoea stops. The medicine also helps relieve fever, cough, and cold. Another preparation is *Balachaturbhadra Churna*, of which 200 mg should be taken daily with honey.

Diet and Other Regimen: The diet of the infant suffering from diarrhoea should consist of milk with less fat. Cow's milk or goat's milk should be given. In case of non-availability of cow's or goat's milk, any milk that is available should be diluted with water.

In some cases, infantile diarrhoea starts because the child may be feeding on the milk of a woman who is pregnant. In such a case, he suffers from a disease known in Ayurveda as *Parigarbhika*. The first step to be taken in such a condition is to switch over to other milk.

The fluid lost through diarrhoea must be replaced immediately with fluid by mouth or an intravenous drip.

Dysentery *(Raktatisar* and *Pravahika)*

Dysentery or bloody flux is a condition characterised by inflammation of the bowels. It is associated with colicky pain in the abdomen, and liquid or semi-solid stools mixed with mucus and blood.

Modern medicine categorises dysentery into two types: bacillary and amoebic.

Causes and Symptoms: Modern medicine believes that both bacillary and amoebic dysentery are caused by infection.

In **bacillary dysentery**, the stool is mixed with blood. Ayurveda terms bacillary dysentery as *Raktatisar*. Many of the remedies prescribed for diarrhoea are useful in treating the bloody flux or bacillary dysentery.

In **amoebic dysentery**, mucus is present in the stools, along with the organism which causes it. In Ayurveda, amoebic dysentery is known as *Pravahika*. Amoebic dysentery is a more serious condition than bacillary dysentery. It is a disease endemic to tropical climates, and once contracted, it may lead to serious complications unless the patient is careful. It is characterised by discharge of mucus in the stools and griping pains in the abdomen. According to Allopathy, the causative organism is *Entamoeba histolytica*. Discharge of mucus, dyspepsia, anaemia, and general weakness are the characteristic symptoms. In more serious cases, the liver may be involved and a condition known as hepatic amoebiasis will arise. Loss of appetite and loss of weight also occur.

Home Remedies: The following home remedies are of use in both bacillary and amoebic dysentery. Lemon juice is efficacious in dealing with ordinary cases of dysentery. A few lemons, peeled and sliced, are added to 250 ml of water and boiled for a few minutes. The strained infusion is administered thrice daily. Small pieces of onions mixed with curd, and given half a dozen times during the day, are also helpful. Equal parts of the tender leaves of the *peepul* tree, coriander leaves, and sugar should be chewed slowly to relieve the condition. Powdered seeds of the *mehandi* (henna) plant mixed with *ghee* should be made into small balls, the size of a betel nut, and taken twice daily with water. The tubercles of *nagarmotha* (nut grass) should be powdered and mixed with fresh ginger and honey. A 20 gm dose of the preparation should be taken thrice daily.

Bael fruit is, perhaps, the most efficacious in the treatment of dysentery of both the varieties. Pulp of the fruit mixed with *gur* should be given thrice daily. For a chronic case of dysentery, unripe *bael* fruit is roasted over the fire and the pulp is mixed with water. Large quantities of the infusion so made should be administered with *gur*. The pulp of the unripe fruit mixed with an equal quantity of dried ginger should be given with buttermilk. The patient should subsist on buttermilk during the course of the treatment.

Medicines & Prescriptions: Chronic cases of **bacillary dysentery** can be cured by administering one tablet of *Kutajaghana Vati* two or three times a day with water or buttermilk before meals. Alternatively, 1 to 2 tablets of *Piyushavalli Rasa* may be taken twice daily with roasted *bael* fruit and *gur.*

For amoebic dysentery, *Kutaja* (*Holarrhena antidysenteria*) is the drug of choice. Powdered bark of the plant is administered thrice daily in one teaspoonful doses. Patients suffering from amoebic dysentery are also liable to suffer from chronic constipation and so, should take two tablespoonfuls of fleaseed husk at bedtime with milk or buttermilk. The Ayurvedic preparation *Rasaparpati* should be given in a dose of 150 mg thrice daily in chronic cases of amoebic dysentery.

Diet and Other Regimen: The patient must live on milk, boiled rice, and sugar. All forms of salt and water should be withheld. As in the case of other diseases, the diet of the patient suffering from either form of dysentery is of the utmost importance. He must avoid fried food, *ghee* and other fats, chillies and condiments, and heavy meals. Meat and its preparations should be avoided except in the case of soups. Fruits with a sour taste like pomegranate, citrus fruits, and *amla* are useful in such cases.

During a severe attack, the patient should be advised complete bedrest. At this stage of the disease, he should even avoid a cold bath.

Gastritis *(Urdhavaga Amlapitta)*

Gastritis or inflammation of the stomach is a troublesome condition which eventually gives rise to many life-threatening complications, if not treated in time.

Causes and Symptoms: The most frequent cause of an attack of gastritis is a dietary indiscretion, such as overeating or excessive intake of alcohol. Infections like influenza, food poisoning, toxins of uraemia and gout, and swallowing of acids and alkalis also give rise to gastritis. Persons having a *pittika* constitution are more prone to geting the disease than others. Constipation tends to aggravate the condition more than any other disorder.

The chief symptoms are: loss of appetite, sickness or nausea, headache, and giddiness. There is also pain and a general feeling of discomfort in the region of the stomach, sour eructations and frequent vomiting—first of food, and then of bilious matter. There is also tenderness in the upper abdomen which is aggravated after the ingestion of food. If the disease becomes chronic, it may lead to anaemia and, consequently, emaciation.

Medicines & Prescriptions: Since the disease is caused by vitiation of *pitta*, the best therapy is purgation in the first instance. Preparations of *ghee* are recommended for treatment of gastritis since it is a substance which counteracts *pitta*. *Sukumara Ghrita* is specific and is administered in doses of one to two teaspoonfuls mixed with a cup of milk and given first thing in the morning. It may lead to some impairment of the digestive powers of the patient in the beginning, but he recovers the power of digestion after some days. *Amalaki* of *amla (Emblica officinalis)* in a powdered form is also helpful; the standard dose is two teaspoonfuls administered four times a day. Alternatively, *Dhatri Lauha* (calx of iron mixed with juice of *amalaki*) should be given in one teaspoonful doses twice daily. In case of persistent constipation in a case of gastritis, *Avipittikara Churna* should be given in a dose of two teaspoonfuls at bed time.

Diet and Other Regimen: The diet should consist of milk with sugar, and a little old rice. Spices and condiments, alcoholic drinks, sour foods, chillies and pungent substances which are likely to aggravate acidity or *pitta* must be avoided. Other substances recommended are: barley, wheat, rice (at least one year old), cucumber, bitter gourd, green banana, pumpkin, pomegranate, and cow's milk.

The patient should not undertake strenuous mental or physical work. Anxiety and anger should be avoided. Bedrest is also advised, but the patient must be encouraged to take a walk of about two kilometres early in the morning.

Ulcers of the Stomach *(Grahani)*

An ulcer is a breach on the surface of the skin or on the membrane lining of any organ such as the stomach. It does not tend to heal quickly. Only those persons who are affected with a *vatika* type of constitution or in whom *vata* is the predominant *dosha* are prone to getting ulcers of the stomach.

Aggravation of the *vata dosha* in the body gives rise to ulcers either in the stomach or the duodenum. The term **peptic ulcer** is a general term applied to all ulcers in the stomach, whereas **duodenal ulcer** is the term applied to an ulcer in the duodenum. The duodenum is the link between the stomach and the jejunum. Pancreatic juice and bile are poured into the duodenum to mix with the permeated food. The duodenum, therefore, plays a major role in the process of digestion.

A duodenal ulcer is a painful disease, the pain being similar to that of colic. The pain comes when the food is being digested. It is probably due to the churning motion of the stomach and ceases when fresh food is ingested. In severe cases of ulcer or when it is too deep, the pain may continue even when there is food in the stomach.

The ulcer results in gradual loss of weight due to impairment of digestion and defective or incomplete absorption of food. Pain makes the patient irritable. The ulcer may bleed, the blood mixing with the stools, or in very severe cases, the blood may come through the mouth. Excessive loss of blood is a serious condition and the patient may have to be hospitalised and given an immediate blood transfusion. Sometimes, there may be only vomiting preceded by eructation, and the patient throwing up the food. But if such an act of vomiting is followed by a rapid and thready pulse which are indications of falling blood pressure, immediate treatment should be given to correct the blood pressure.

Medicines & Prescriptions: The Ayurvedic medicine of choice in gastric ulcers is *Sukumara Ghrita*. It should be administered in doses of two teaspoonfuls with warm milk on an empty stomach. If the patient is unable to digest *ghee,* or if *ghee* does not agree with him, the medicine should be given with warm water. The dose must be adjusted according to the digestive powers of the patient. Some patients are unable to tolerate standard doses of the medicine and the dose must, therefore, be altered according to the patient's condition. The dose should gradually be increased to six teaspoonfuls a day.

The pain of the ulcer is best controlled with another preparation--*Shankha Bhasma.* In the case of excruciating pain, *Maha Shankha Vati* should be given.

Ulcers in the stomach or the duodenum may heal by themselves. Any disturbance in the routine of the patient may, however, aggravate them again. The remedy mentioned above should, therefore, be taken for a long time. The subsidence of the colic should not be taken as the end of the malady. Medication should continue for some weeks after the pain has totally vanished.

Diet and Other Regimen: Since hyperacidity or *Amlapitta* is the villain of the piece which ultimately leads to stomach ulcers, the first step is to withhold all foods which aggravate the condition. Fried foods and spices, specially chillies, should be totally prohibited. Bland, easily-digestible foods should be the mainstay of the patient's diet. Milk should be freely taken, preferably at intervals of three to four hours during the day, because the pain of the ulcer occurs at times when the stomach is empty. Milk, wheat, and *ghee* should be taken in adequate quantities.

In addition to the diet prescribed above, the patient must be advised to keep himself free from worry and stresses of life which are likely to exacerbate the ulcer pain. He must take sufficient rest and sleep for an hour or so during the day. His bowel movement must be ensured because constipation can only contribute to worsening of the condition. The best way to deal with constipation of patients suffering from gastric ulcers is either husk of fleaseed taken at bedtime or castor oil. No strong purgatives should be administered to such patients.

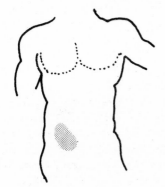

Appendicitis

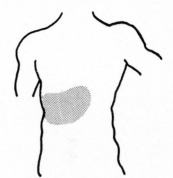

Inflammation of the Liver

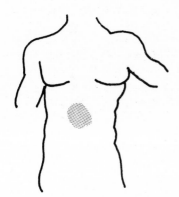

Stomach Ulcer

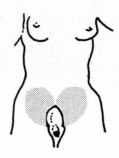

Ovarian Tumour

Pain in the Abdomen
Pain is present in the shaded areas

Colic Pain *(Parinama Shula)*

The term colic is generally applied to pain in the abdomen, usually around the umbilicus or navel. It comes in spasms and is generally associated with constipation. Simple colic commonly arises from the presence of some indigestible matter in the alimentary canal. Colic pain is not accompanied by fever, which distinguishes it from colitis—the inflammation of the intestine.

According to Ayurveda, colic in adults is either due to presence of wind in the stomach, the result of chronic constipation, or a result of exposure to damp and cold. Infants who are being artificially fed are also prone to this condition.

Colic pain may also be due to appendicitis, gallstones or stones in the kidney, inflammation of the liver or the ovaries. In Ayurveda, it is known as *Shula* and is caused by the aggravation of *vayu*, one of the three dominant *doshas*.

Colic pain may also travel to other parts of the body like the shoulder blades or the genital organs. It may also be accompanied by nausea and vomiting.

Medicines & Prescriptions: Immediate relief to the victim of colic can be provided by administration of two remedies: *Shankha Bhasma* or *Hingvashtaka Churna*, the drugs of choice in Ayurveda for colic pain. In severe cases, *Maha Shankha Vati* should be administered in doses of two tablets, four times a day. Another drug is *Lahsunaadi Vati* which should be given in a dose of two tablets, four times a day. *Abhraka Bhasma* can also be given in doses of 150 mg, mixed with honey, four times a day.

After providing relief for the initial colic pain, the wise physician must cure the causes of the disease, because pain is usually an indication of a disease rather than a disease in itself. If the colic is due to appendicitis or presence of stones in the kidney or the bladder, steps should be taken to relieve those conditions. But if the pain is caused by the presence of *vata*, it should be taken to mean that chronic constipation or dyspepsia has caused it. In that case, steps should be taken to relieve constipation after the attack of colic has passed. A mild purgative should be given after which the patient should be advised to change his diet. In other words, he should take foods which do not aggravate the constipation.

Diet and Other Regimen: Fried foods, carbohydrates, and starch should be restricted to the minimum. Boiled vegetables and fruits should be taken in larger quantities and fats should be avoided.

Regular habits of eating and defecation are helpful. Morning walks or exercise are recommended.

Intestinal Worms

Intestinal worms give rise to many symptoms which are troublesome and which may lead to severe complications. The most common parasites found in human intestines are: round worms, tape worms, hook worms, thread worms, and giardia.

Causes and Symptoms: The presence of such parasites in the intestines gives rise to symptoms such as a voracious appetite, diarrhoea, anaemia, and headache. Thread worms give rise to acute irritation round the anus, forcing the sufferer to scratch it. Round worms may cause cough, vomiting, nausea, and loss of appetite. Hook worms may lead to anaemia, since these parasites tend to suck the blood of the sufferer.

The worms are passed out with the stools. In insanitary conditions, the worms are likely to spread and cause further infestation to others. Continued presence of worms may lead to obstruction of the intestine or the bile ducts, giving rise to further complications.

Home Remedies: Seeds of fresh ripe papaya, administered in 5 to 10 gm doses with water are an excellent remedy for intestinal worms. Other anthelminthics (drugs which destroy intestinal worms) are fresh seeds of *palash* (flame of the forest), *vidanga* (*Embelia ribes*), or *baheda*, one of the *triphalas*. Tender leaves of the Indian coral, *mandar*, given with honey are also helpful. *Vidanga* and *palash* seeds ground together should be administered in one teaspoonful doses thrice daily. *Haridra* (*Curcuma longa*) is also helpful if the powder of the rhizome of this plant is given in a dose of one teaspoonful, three times a day, with a cup of milk. This drug is also useful in urticaria and fevers which may be associated with intestinal worms. Raw areca nut should be ground on a piece of stone and mixed with the juice of a lime. It destroys thread worms more effectively than any other remedies. Seeds of round bitter gourd (*tumbi*), in a quantity of 200 mg, taken with buttermilk, will deal with the most intractable case of intestinal worms.

Medicines & Prescriptions: About 200 mg of *Khurasani Ajwain* in powdered form should be administered after the patient has eaten about 10 gm of *gur*. The drug is available in the form of thymol and is specific for round worms.

Other specific drugs are *Kamipallak Churna* in doses of 1–2 gms, and *Kirmani Ajwain Churna* in doses of 1–3 gms, to be taken thrice daily.

Diet and Other Regimen: The treatment for worms must start with the diet. The patient should be kept on a light diet; heavy, not readily-digested foods should be withheld. Sweet things are also best avoided because they help the gut to turn into a breeding ground for worms. Thread worms, it may be stated, trouble infants more than adults, because their mainstay is milk or sweets and there are no bitter or pungent substances in the diet of infants. Older patients must be encouraged to include bitter things in their food, such as bitter gourd (*karela*), *neem* flowers, and a bitter variety of drumsticks. Garlic should be added in substantial quantities to the vegetables or meats eaten by the patients suffering from intestinal worms.

If there is constipation in addition to intestinal worms, purgatives should be used. The patient should never suppress the urge to evacuate his bowels. Fasting for at least one day in the week is also helpful in controlling intestinal worms.

Piles *(Arsha)*

Piles or haemorrhoids consist of a varicose and, often, inflamed condition of the veins around the anal canal.

Causes and Symptoms: A person suffers from piles when the veins in the anal region become varicosed. The prime cause of piles is constipation, the others being a sedentary way of life, lack of exercise, and some morbid conditions of the liver.

Piles are of two types: **dry piles**, in which there is inflammation of the external piles, and pain which may continue all the time, becoming unbearable at the time of voiding the bowels; and **bleeding piles**, in which the internal piles start bleeding. In the latter type of piles, there may be excessive bleeding, leading to anaemia and consequent emaciation.

If piles are neglected, they may lead to prolapse of the rectum, in which the rectum protrudes out of its casing; impotence; proctitis or inflammation of the rectum; and haemorrhage. Excessive bleeding from piles may, in some cases, lead to death due to loss of blood.

Medicines & Prescriptions: Sushruta has advocated surgery for curing piles, but Charaka, the physician, has advised drug therapy. Ayurveda has recommended the use of drugs to increase the digestive powers, to relieve constipation, and to relieve flatulence which exacerbates the pain of piles. In the case of bleeding piles, the drug of choice is *Nagakesara* (*Mesua ferrea*). The powder of the flower of this plant should be administered to the patient in one teaspoonful doses, thrice daily. *Haritaki* (*Terminalia chebula*) is recommended when there is bleeding, as well as inflammation and pain. One teaspoonful, given two to three times a day with milk, is sure to relieve the condition.

Chirabilvadikashay, Lavanottamadi Churna, Samashara Churna, Nagkesharayoga, and *Samangadi Churna* are some of the other standard Ayurvedic remedies for both dry and bleeding piles. These may be taken according to prescribed dosages.

Diet and Other Regimen: The patient's food should consist of a bland diet and foods which are easily digestible. Goat's milk is also helpful in this condition.

The patient should be advised not to use a hard seat or ride horses during the course of treatment. He should not indulge in too much sex, nor suppress the urge to void the stools for fear of pain which accompanies dry piles.

Metabolism & Disorders of the Endocrine Glands

रममांसप्रमाणरत् रमसंहननो नरः ।
दृढेन्द्रियो विकाराणां न बलेनाभिभूयते ॥

Persons with a proportionate muscular structure and compactness of the body, no doubt, possess very strong sensory and motor organs and, as such, they are not overcome by the onslaught of disease.

CHARAKA SAMHITA

METABOLISM IS a series of complex processes by which the human body converts food, water, and oxygen into tissue, energy, and waste products. It is a continuous process and goes on in every cell of the body. It comprises the breaking down of substances into simpler parts, and their shuffling and recombination into countless new substances that compose the body. For example, the carbohydrates are broken down by enzymes and acids and converted into pure sugar or glucose.

The constructive chemical and physical process by which food materials are adapted for the use of the body is known as anabolism; and the destructive process by which energy is produced with the breaking down of tissues into waste products is called catabolism. The two processes together are called metabolism.

Basal metabolism or the basal metabolic rate is the rate at which energy is consumed when a person is at complete rest. When a person is placed in a state of complete rest, the metabolic rate can be measured by measuring the amounts of oxygen and carbon dioxide exchanged during breathing under certain standard conditions. The BMR (Basal Metabolic Rate) is an index of a person's health.

Metabolism is controlled by the endocrine glands--a term applied to certain organs whose function is to secrete into the blood or lymph, a substance which plays an important role in relation to general chemical changes or to the activities of the other organs at a distance. Some organs have a double function, such as the pancreas, which pours digestive secretions from a duct into the intestine, and, at the same time, has an endocrine or hormone secretion which is absorbed into the blood. Defects in the secretions of the various glands give rise to many diseases.

The chief endocrine glands are the thyroid gland, adrenal glands, pituitary body, parathyroid glands, pancreas, ovaries, and the testes. A balancing act exists between different endocrine glands. For example, secretion of the adrenal glands controls the action of the pancreatic secretion. Other glands

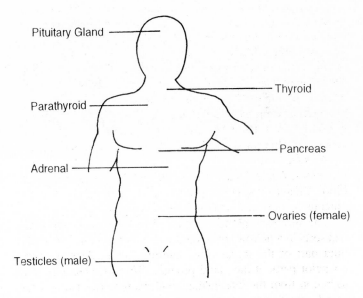

Endocrine Glands

have an associated action; for example, the extract of the pituitary gland stimulates the production of normal secretion of the thyroid. During healthy bodily activity, there appears to be a constant state of balancing among the different endocrine secretions.

The **thyroid gland** is situated in the front of the neck and produces a secretion which plays a very important role in regulating the general metabolism of the body. When it is defective, the conditions known as myxoedema (in adults) and cretinism (in children) result. An excess of its secretion is associated with a condition known as exophthalmic goitre or thyrotoxicosis.

The **adrenal glands**, also known as suprarenal glands, lie above the upper part of the kidneys. The central portion of the glands secretes adrenaline and noradrenaline. The moment a person faces a situation of danger or shock, the glands become active and secrete adrenaline into the blood stream. The blood vessels are constricted, and the arteries of the muscles and the coronary arteries are dilated. The systolic blood pressure rises, as does the blood sugar level. This raises the metabolic rate and leads to a diminution of muscle fatigue. That is why a person is able to perform functions which he would be totally unable to do under normal circumstances. Malfunctioning of the adrenal glands leads to a disease called Addison's disease. The secretion of the glands, namely, adrenaline, is now synthetically prepared and is used extensively in modern medicine in 1:1000 solution for checking bleeding and providing relief for an asthmatic attack, or anaphylactic shock.

As stated earlier, if the adrenal glands fail to produce their secretions, Addison's disease results and there is anaemia, low blood pressure, wasting, pigmentation of the skin and the mucous membranes, and subnormal temperature.

The **pituitary gland** is attached to the base of the brain and rests in a hollow space on the base of the skull, above the hind part of the throat. The anterior, intermediate, and the posterior parts of the gland produce different secretions. The secretion from the intermediate and the posterior parts of the gland contributes greatly to stimulating the contractions of smooth muscle, such as the muscles of the uterus, intestine, and the blood vessels. The anterior part of the gland secretes hormones which stimulate growth, development of sex, secretion of milk, and also exert a controlling influence on most of the other endocrine glands. It is in this sense that the pituitary gland is called the master gland and its malfunctioning can accelerate the deterioration of almost all bodily functions.

The **parathyroid glands** are four minute bodies lying at the side of, or behind the thyroid gland. They help in controlling the absorption of calcium by the bones and other tissues. Defective functioning of the glands results in tetany or spasm of muscles.

The **pancreas** is another endocrine gland situated in the upper part of the abdomen, and in addition to the digestive enzymes, it produces a hormone known as insulin. This helps in adapting sugary foods for incorporation in the muscles and other tissues that particularly require such foodstuffs. A malfunctioning of the pancreas results in diabetes mellitus in which sugar is not absorbed into the cells and tends to accumulate in the blood, and is then excreted through the urine.

The **ovaries** and the **testes** are the glands which, in addition to their main function of producing reproductive cells, secrete substances which have a general effect upon the other bodily functions.

The ovaries secrete at least two hormones, which help in the fertilisation of the ovum by the sperm. Their malfunctioning results in sterility in women. The testes secrete a hormone known as testosterone which is responsible for the growth of the male secondary sex organs. The failure to secrete this hormone results in male sterility and impotence.

Disorders of the Thyroid Gland

The hormone of the thyroid gland—thyroxine—is one of the most important controls of metabolism in the body. If the secretion is deficient in children, they develop a condition known as cretinism, which is a failure to grow. If the deficiency develops in adult life, the individual becomes obese, lethargic, and develops a coarse skin—a condition known as myxoedema. Overactivity of the thyroid or hyperthyroidism results in loss of weight, rapid heart rate, and a highly strung nervous temperament. The condition known as exophthalmic goitre, thyroitoxicosis, or Grave's disease, is practically the same as hyperthyroidism, but, in certain cases at least, there is evidence to suggest that not only is the output of the secretion of the thyroid increased, but there is some abnormality in it. The most common disorder of the thyroid gland is goitre.

Goitre *(Galaganda)*

Goitre is of two types: simple goitre and exophthalmic goitre. In the latter the eyeballs protrude from their sockets.

Causes and Symptoms: Allopathy believes that simple goitre is caused by the lack of iodine in drinking water. The belief is based on the observation that it is endemic to certain areas where the water supply is deficient in iodine. But according to Ayurveda, goitre is the result of aggravation of *kapha* and diminution of *pitta*, which then lead to vitiation of *mamsa* and *meda dhatus*.

In simple goitre, there is a swelling in the neck region which is well marked. Excessive growth may cause discomfort, and even lead to serious symptoms from its pressure on the wind pipe, the food pipe, and other parts of the neck.

Medicines & Prescriptions: Goitre can be cured by the administration of *kanchanara (Bauhinia variegata)*. The bark of the tree is given in the form of a decoction. An ounce of the decoction is given twice daily on an empty stomach. A compound preparation, *Kanchanara Guggulu,* is recommended in a dose of one tablet, twice daily. The dose can be increased according to the severity of the disease. The ideal dose is four tablets, three times a day, followed by milk or water.

A standard Ayurvedic preparation, *Amritadhaya Taila*, should be given in two daily doses of 11 gm each.

Home Remedies: A fine paste made of the vegetable *jalakumbhi (Pistia straticies)* applied over the affected part helps in reducing the swelling. The juice obtained from the *jalakumbhi* should be given in doses of 11 to 22 gm a day. It increases the amount of iodine, the lack of which, according to Allopathy, is one of the factors responsible for the disease.

Diet and Other Regimen: According to Charaka, goitre does not strike those who take milk in adequate quantities. In addition, old rice, barley, *moong* dal, Bengal gram, cucumber, sugar juice, and milk products are recommended for a goitre patient. Sour and heavy substances are contraindicated.

Exercises of the neck are also recommended.

Diabetes Mellitus *(Madhumeha)*

Diabetes Mellitus is a condition in which there is faulty carbohydrate metabolism. It is one of the most serious disorders of the metabolism, and if left undiagnosed or untreated, it may lead to rapid emaciation and ultimately death.

Causes and Symptoms: The disease is generally hereditary and people with a defective diet are more susceptible to it than others. People whose diet consists mainly of carbohydrates, those who are fat, and those who lead a sedentary life, are more prone to fall a victim to it than others. Diabetes is of two types: juvenile onset; maturity onset.

Diabetes mellitus is due to decreased secretion of insulin from the pancreas, which normally helps in the transfer of glucose from the blood to the cells, in the absence of which, sugar accumulates in the blood and is not converted into energy as it should. The onset of the disease is gradual and, sometimes, it is too late for it to be controlled. The first symptoms are reduced body strength and loss of weight. The urine output goes up from its normal quantity of two to three pints to ten or twenty in twenty-four hours. The sugar passed through the urine may increase. The amount of sugar in the blood increases after a meal instead of being absorbed into the system. A troublesome symptom is excessive thirst. A diabetic takes more and more liquids and passes more and more urine, leading to loss of sugar which should have been assimilated into the system. The diabetic also has a voracious appetite, but in spite of the large amounts of food that he takes, he goes on losing strength and weight. Poor vitality of the tissues caused by the lack of absorption of sugar leads to various complications like skin eruptions. There is intense itching in the groins and eczema on various parts of the body. Sometimes, there is a tendency of getting gangrene in the lower extremities and any injury sustained by the patient is difficult to heal.

As a rule, diabetes advances comparatively slowly except in the case of young people, in whom its progress is likely to be very rapid. The younger the patient, the swifter is the course of the disease. Dimness of vision, cataract, weakness and pain in the limbs, and inflammatory chest diseases may develop. Occasionally, death occurs due to exhaustion or from the condition known as diabetic coma.

Home Remedies: The age-old nostrum of taking two tender leaves of *neem* and *bilva* each, on an empty stomach in the morning, has been found helpful in reducing the blood sugar. Rose apple (*jamun*) is another fruit which controls diabetes.

The second step before medication is to control the amount of food that the diabetic takes. If he is overweight, a strict regimen of diet should be initiated to bring down his body weight. Juice of the leaves of the bitter gourd plant and its fruit should be administered in doses of one ounce twice daily, preferably on an empty stomach. Seeds of bitter gourd may be ground and taken with food. *Shilajit* is another medicine which has an anti-diabetic effect.

Medicines & Prescriptions: A standard Ayurvedic preparation, *Vasanta Kusumakara*, is particularly favoured by the practitioners. Two grains of the preparation are mixed with half a teaspoon of cream and one-fourth teaspoon of sugar, and given twice daily on an empty stomach. Other remedies are:

1. *Chandraprabha Vati.*	500 mg of the medicine should be mixed with juice of *karela* or stone of rose apple and given thrice daily.
2. *Shilajita;* *Nyagrodadhi Churna.*	240 mg of *Shilajita* and 3 gm of *Nyagrodadhi Churna* should be taken twice daily with decoction of *arni* after meals.

180

3. *Vasantakusumakara Rasa;* *Shuddha Shilajit.*	120 mg of *Vasanta-kusumakara Rasa* and 240 mg of *Shuddha Shilajit* to be taken twice daily with rose apple stones.
4. *Nag Bhasma; Haldi; Amalaki Churna.*	120 mg of *Nag Bhasma,* and 500 mg each of *Haldi* and *Amalaki Churna* to be taken twice daily with honey.

Diet and Other Regimen: The most important step in the treatment of diabetes, once it is confirmed by the examination of the urine and blood of the patient, is the restriction of diet of the patient. All sugary substances and those containing carbohydrates should be restricted. Sugar in any form, rice, potatoes, sweet fruits (except rose apple—*jamun*), and refined wheat flour should be taken sparingly. Fat intake should also be reduced, particularly that of *ghee* or butter. A little oil may be taken without any harm.

Vegetables like *karela*—bitter gourd, drumsticks, and *bimbi* are particularly recommended. Bitter gourd has a medicinal property of helping assimilation of carbohydrates into the cells. This was confirmed by a UK research team some years ago. The vegetable has the property of reactivating the pancreas.

A diabetic should be asked to take light exercise and not sleep during the day. A yogic exercise, *Matsyendrasana*, is particularly useful in checking the severity of the disease. The sufferer should be careful to avoid injuries because the inability of his system to absorb sugar reduces his capacity to heal a wound. The slow healing process may even lead to gangrene of the affected part.

Obesity *(Medoroga)*

It is not easy to define the state of obesity except in very broad terms. It is, generally speaking, a condition of the body characterised by excessive accumulation of fat under the skin and around certain internal organs. The weight charts for men and women according to their heights are only rough indications of the state of health of a person depending on his body weight. Readers must have come across persons whom they thought to be fat but who were quite active and healthy, and did not suffer from the disorders which are commonly associated with obesity.

Causes and Symptoms: Various causes are assigned to the development of obesity. It may be due to disturbances of some of the endocrine glands, such as the thyroid, pituitary, and the sex glands. Obesity runs in some families. But beyond that, obesity is due to wrong diet and, generally, overeating. A luxurious, inactive, or sedentary life is a well-recognised predisposing factor. The more immediate exciting causes are over-feeding and intake of liquids, particularly alcoholic beverages or liquors. Intake of food beyond the quantities required to replace the energy lost, goes towards increasing the fat in the body.

Good health cannot be maintained for long under conditions of excessive obesity, for the increase in the bulk of the body, rendering exercise more difficult, leads to relaxation and defective nutrition of muscles, while the accumulation of fat in the chest and abdomen causes serious embarrassment to the functioning of various organs in these cavities. In general, the mental activity of the highly corpulent becomes impaired. The obese are more liable to fall prey to many diseases because of lowered body resistance. According to Ayurveda, obesity is caused by the impairment of the *Agni* responsible for the break up of the molecules of fat.

Medicines & Prescriptions: The following medicines, if taken over a long period, along with a restricted diet and increased exercise of the body, would definitely help in reducing body fat.

The basic purpose of Ayurvedic medication is to strengthen the *agni* by administration of drugs like *Guggulu, Sunthi, Pippali,* and *Maricha. Guggulu (Balasmodendron mukul)* is the drug of choice in obesity. Fifteen grains of purified *Guggulu* should be administered four times a day, followed by hot water or any other hot drink, preferably skimmed milk.

Haritaki is another useful drug which not only clears the bowels but also helps in reducing the amount of fat in the body. The pulp of this fruit should be given in doses of one teaspoonful at bedtime with hot water.

The following prescriptions are also recommended for the obese:

1. *Triyushanadi Lauha; Navaka Guggulu; Trikatu Churna.*	240 mg of *Triyushanadi Lauha,* and 1 gm each of *Nayaka Guggulu* and *Trikatu Churna* should be taken thrice daily with cold decoction of *triphala* and a little honey.
2. *Lauharishta.*	24 ml should be taken twice daily, after meals, with lukewarm water.
3. *Arogyavardhini.*	240 mg to be taken thrice daily with decoction of *haritaki.*

Diet and Other Regimen: The most important requisite is to reduce the intake of food and to increase the output or expenditure of energy through controlled regimen of exercise.

If the intake of food is more than the quantity required, fat tends to accumulate and leads to distressing symptoms associated with obesity.

Green vegetables and salads, fruit juices, and a liquid diet are best for a fat person. The intake of fat and carbohydrates should be severely restricted. Foods with large bulk but comparatively less nutrition should be recommended. The total calorie intake should be reduced.

In addition to reduction of diet, the patient should be advised to give up sedentary habits and to take exercise. Sleeping during the day, reclining on sofas and soft chairs, and a lethargic way of life should be given up.

Gout *(Vatarakta)*

Gout, according to Ayurveda, is another disorder of the metabolism which has afflicted mankind since the dawn of recorded history. The disorder is associated with the presence

183

of large amounts of uric acid in the blood, manifesting itself by inflammation of the joints, with deposition therein of urate of soda, and also by morbid changes in various important organs. Uric acid is formed during the metabolism of proteins and is excreted through the kidneys. The amount of uric acid found in patients suffering from gout is always above the normal level, that is, more than 0.5 mg/100 ml.

Causes and Symptoms: Gout is, to a marked degree, hereditary. In 50 to 80 per cent of the cases of gout, family history is present. It attacks sedentary people more readily than the active. Inadequate exercise, a rich diet, habitual overindulgence in animal foods and rich dishes, and alcohol are important precipitating factors, even though teetotallers and vegetarians are not immune to the disease. It is more common in mature age than in the earlier years of life, and men are more susceptible to it than women, among whom the disorder may appear after menopause.

An attack of gout may appear without warning, or there may be premonitory symptoms like feeble and capricious appetite, flatulence, uneasiness in the right side of the region of the liver, and irritation in the urinary organs. Various forms of nervous disturbances are also present in the form of extreme irritation, numbness, and coldness in the limbs. On the night of the attack, the patient retires to rest apparently quite well, but at about two or three o'clock in the morning, he is awakened by a painful feeling in the foot, most commonly in the big toe, or in the instep of the heal. With the pain there is often a distinct shivering and feverishness. The pain soon becomes agonising.

The big toe is generally inflamed and is of deep red colour. There may also be pitting over the surface if it is pressed. The patient is extremely uncomfortable during the attack, which is followed by dyspepsia, thirst, constipation, and cramps in the limbs. If the disease is left untreated, it may spread to other joints. According to Ayurveda, the disease is the result of the vitiation of *vata*. Intake of mutually contradictory foods and failure of the body to excrete the wastes from the body ultimately leads to a serious case of gout.

Medicines and Prescriptions: *Panchatikta Ghrita Guggulu* is the first drug of choice in dealing with a case of gout. Two teaspoonfuls of it, mixed with warm milk, should be given twice daily on an empty stomach for the first fortnight. *Guduchyadi Taila* or *Pinda Taila* should be applied to the affected part.

When the acute symptoms are relieved, the above medication should be followed by a course of *Kaishora Guggulu*--five tablets, three times a day for a week or so. This should be followed by two ounces of decoction of *Manjishtha (Rubia cardifolia)*.

Decoction of the root bark of *Ashvattha (Ficus riligosa)* given in two ounce doses once a day helps the patient to throw off the effects of gout.

Diet and Other Regimen: Fried foods, sour substances like curds, fatty substances, and alcohol should be avoided. Old rice, wheat, *moong* dal, meat soup, garlic, onions, bitter gourd, papaya, and green banana are helpful in this condition.

The patient should avoid exposure to cold, cold baths, and heavy exercise. Care should be taken to see that the patient is not constipated. A mild laxative, *haritaki,* may be given in a two teaspoonful dose at bedtime with warm water.

Diseases of the Urinary and Reproductive System

शकृतरुत् प्रतीष्याता द्वार्यविंगुणतां गत: ।
आध्मानं वातशूलभ च मूत्रकृच्छ्रं करोति च ॥

Interruption of excretion of waste products leads to vitiation of vayu, pain, and dysuria.

BHOJARATNAKAR

THE KIDNEYS are a pair of excretory organs, situated on either side of the vertebral column, in the upper posterior part of the abdomen. They are grouped under the most important parts of the body, and any malfunctioning in them can lead to serious disorders and, sometimes, death. Renal failure, which is the incapacity of the kidneys to perform their function, is one of the most serious ailments to which humans are susceptible.

The chief function of the kidneys is to filter the blood and to remove its impurities which are excreted through the urine. The blood passes through the glomeruli, a bunch of small capillaries with capsules, which filter the non-protein portion of the plasma. The efficiency of and the burden on the kidneys can be judged from the fact that in humans, they filter between 150 to 200 litres of plasma in 24 hours. The usable portion of the blood is returned to the heart through the renal vein. The waste matter is ejected through the urinary bladder. Substances like amino-acids, glucose, sodium, potassium, calcium, magnesium, and chlorine are reabsorbed into the system and urea, uric acid, and phosphates are excreted.

186

Diseases of the Kidneys

When the kidneys are diseased, their functioning is impaired, and impurities which should have been excreted, continue to remain in the system, poisoning it. The general term used to describe the accumulation of poisons is uraemia.

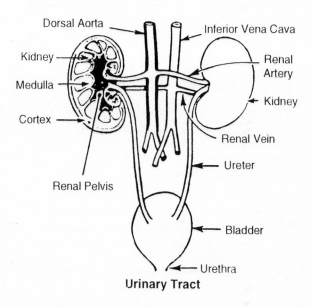

Urinary Tract

The following are the symptoms common to the various types of kidney diseases:

Pain: Inflammation of the kidney and formation of calculi or stones in the kidneys produce pain in the renal region. The pain of inflammation is situated high up in the loins, but the pain in the back, generally referred to as renal colic, is usually a symptom of formation of stones in the kidney and UTI (urinary tract infection). It is of a very agonising nature and leaves the sufferer prostrate even after it has passed.

Urine: The urine almost invariably shows the changes in kidney diseases. The quantity diminishes in acute conditions and may even contain blood. If there are traces of pus in the urine, it might indicate suppuration of the diseased kidneys. In the case of stones, urine examination would show the presence of deposits of the substances of which the stones are made. In Bright's disease, a chronic kidney condition, there is excess of albumin found in the urine.

Dropsy: Another cardinal symptom of kidney malfunctioning is the presence of dropsy, which is an abnormal collection of fluid under the skin, particularly around the eyes, especially in the morning.

Changes in Circulation of Blood: Changes in circulation of blood take place in chronic kidney diseases like pyelonephritis which leave an abnormal amount of uric acid in the blood, giving rise to high blood pressure. There is also thickening of the arteries as in Bright's disease, leading to pain in the chest, loss of mental power, breathlessness, impairment of vision, and even apoplexy.

Uraemia: Uraemia is a condition in which there is a general poisoning of the system due to the failure of the kidneys to expel the waste matter, that is, urea.

Dysuria *(Mutrakrichha)*

Dysuria is a condition in which urine is expelled painfully and in small amounts every time.

Causes and Symptoms: A patient suffering from dysuria may always feel the urge to urinate, but may not be able to get satisfaction from the act of urination. The feeling of relief which comes to a healthy person is missing in a patient suffering from dysuria.

The four main causes of dysuria according to Allopathy are: cystitis or inflammation of the bladder; inflammation of the urethra; venereal diseases like gonorrhoea[1]; and, sometimes, an enlarged prostrate gland. Excessive amount of acid present in the urine also seems to produce the feeling of pain in the process of its excretion from the system.

---

1. Dysuria relating to syphilis and gonorrhoea is discussed under those diseases.

Ayurveda recognises eight types of dysuria: three caused by the vitiation of the different *doshas* of the body; one caused by the vitiation of all the three *doshas*; one caused by the failure of the system in ejecting the waste matter; and the others by the presence of stones in the bladder.

The cardinal symptoms of dysuria as described above are: scanty urine; pain during the act of urination; pain in the penis in men, and in women in the lower abdomen; urine mixed with blood; feeling of heaviness in the renal region and the scrotum; and the ever-present urge to pass urine.

If dysuria is caused by the presence of stones in the kidney or the bladder, it is of *vata* origin, because the vitiation of *vayu* leads to the accumulation of biochemical substances around the nucleus of urinary salts, which take the shape of stones.

Medicines & Prescriptions: *Pashanabheda (Bergenia ligulata)* is the drug of choice for the treatment of stones in the kidney or the bladder, because unless that condition is treated, dysuria caused by it cannot be relieved. One teaspoonful of the powder of the root of this drug is given thrice daily. A decoction of the drug may also be given in 50 ml doses, thrice daily.

Decoction of the bark of the *varuna (Cretiva religiosa)* tree is also useful in dealing with this condition. In case urine is obstructed by a stone in the urinary tract, *Gokshuradi Guggulu* is the drug of choice. But the most important drug used for this condition is *Shilajit*, followed by the compound preparation *Chandraprabha Vati*. Other prescriptions for painful or scanty urine are:

1. *Eladi Churna; Shweta Parpati; Yavakshara.*	1 gm each of *Eladi Churna* and *Shweta Parpati*, and 1/2 gm of *Yavakshara* to be taken four times daily with decoction of *Pashanabhedada.*
2. *Mutrakrichhakantaka Rasa; Shweta Parpati.*	240 mg of *Mutrakrichhakantaka Rasa* and 2 gm of *Shweta Parpati* to be taken with *Amritadi Quath* six times daily.

If dysuria is due to vitiation of *pitta* or *kapha*, the following drugs should be administered:

1. *Trinetra Rasa;*
   Chandrakala Rasa;
   Sheetala Parpati.

   240 mg each of *Trinetra Rasa* and *Chandrakala Rasa*, and 2 gm of *Sheetala Parpati* to be taken thrice daily with *Trinapanchamula Quath.*

2. *Khasoraka Yoga;*
   Varundya Lauha;
   Powder of Cardamom Seeds.

   240 mg of *Khasoraka Yoga*, and 500 mg each of *Varundya Lauha* and powder of cardamom seeds to be taken thrice daily with honey.

3. *Mutrakrichhantaka Rasa;*
   Varitara Lauha Bhasma.

   240 mg of *Mutrakrichhantaka Rasa* and 120 mg of *Varitara Lauha Bhasma* to be taken thrice daily with honey.

4. *Shalajita;*
   Powder of Cardamom Seeds.

   500 mg each of *Shalajita* and powder of cardamom seeds to be taken thrice daily with honey.

In case there is discharge of blood with the urine, the following prescription is the best:

Rasa Sindura;
Honey or Trikantakadya Ghrita.

120 mg of *Rasa Sindura* and 10 gm of honey or *Trikantakadya Ghrita* to be taken thrice daily.

Home Remedies: In addition to the medicines, fomentation of the renal region with a hot water bag is indicated in most cases of dysuria. The affected area may also be coated with the following substances: droppings of mice mascerated with water; ear wax of a buffalo; equal quantities of saltpetre and pulp of root of banana tree.

Ayurveda has given the name *mutrakrichha,* and allopathy—dysuria, to diseases of the kidneys whose cardinal symptom is difficulty or pain during the act of urination. Most of the diseases of the kidneys, known variously as Bright's disease, nephritis, albuminuria, formation of stones in the kidneys or the urinary tract, in which the chief symptom is dysuria, can be cured through the use of treatment mentioned above. Only in the case of venereal diseases like gonorrhoea, which also exhibit the symptoms of dysuria, is the treatment different. In case of obstruction of urine caused by gonorrhoea, the physician should first treat that malady before any relief from painful urination can be expected.

Diet and Other Regimen: The patient suffering from dysuria should be advised to refrain from eating beans and pulses. The white variety of pumpkin and gourds are useful for this condition. Green vegetables like spinach, tomatoes, and ladies' fingers should be avoided.

The patient should be asked to give up a sedentary lifestyle and take walks. Constipation should be avoided through a proper diet, but if it occurs, mild laxatives should be used. The intake of liquids, particularly water, should be increased.

Haematuria (*Adhoga Raktapitta*)

Haematuria is a condition in which there is blood in the urine.

Causes and Symptoms: The blood in the urine may come from any part of the urinary tract, including the bladder. Haematuria is sometimes found in cystitis or inflammation of the bladder. Inflammation of the kidneys due to Bright's disease may also, in some cases, lead to haematuria. The presence of blood in the urine gives it a brownish or smoky colour. Another condition leading to haematuria is the presence of stones in the urinary tract. Sometimes, when the stone moves with the flow of the discharge, it tends to scratch the urethra which produces blood. The difference is merely, that in case of the scratching of the urethra, the blood will be of bright colour; if the blood is from the bladder or the kidneys, the urine will have a brownish hue.

Ayurveda treats haematuria as a variety of *Adhoga Raktapitta,* that is, the downward vitiation of the *pitta* in blood.

In severe cases of this malady, the patient may be found to be passing blood in place of urine.

Medicines and Prescriptions: *Goksura* (*Tribulus rerrestris*) is the drug of choice for this condition. Powder of the seed of the drug is administered in one teaspoonful doses twice a day. It should be taken with honey for better results. Another drug which is highly effective in this case is *Silajatu*. It should be given in one teaspoonful doses with milk, twice a day.

Diet and Other Regimen: The diet recommended for patients of haematuria comprises vegetables such as bitter gourd and drumsticks. Hot and spicy foods should be avoided; meat soups may be given in moderate quantities. The juice of white pumpkin mixed with sugarcane juice helps towards a faster recovery. Pomegranate and *amla* are useful in any form.

The patient should be advised to desist from sexual intercourse during the course of the treatment. The intake of liquids, particularly water, should be increased. Alcohol and other drinks should be avoided.

Enlargement of the Prostate Gland (*Mutraghata*)

Dysuria may be caused by the enlargement of the prostate gland too, in which case, it is known as *Mutraghata* in Ayurveda. In this condition, the urine cannot be properly voided through the urethra.

The prostate gland lies at the neck of the bladder in men and surrounds that part of the urethra lying within it. The gland is of importance because, in late life, it is apt to increase in size and change in shape in such a way as to obstruct the flow of urine from the bladder. There is great difficulty in passing urine and the patient strains himself without voiding the urine. Or, it may come in drops, leaving the sufferer always with the desire of voiding urine. Modern medicine takes recourse to surgery to ameliorate the condition. In most cases, the gland is removed since it is one of the common sites of cancer. Obstruction of urine caused in this condition may be of many types depending on the *dosha* which has been vitiated. There may be spasmodic stricture of the urethra, distension of the bladder, or inflammation of the bladder or the urethra—conditions generally accompanying enlargement of the prostate.

Medicines and Prescriptions: In most cases of enlargement of the prostate gland, the medicines indicated for dysuria are to be given. The doses may be increased according to the severity of the condition.

A quick remedy is to give 50 ml juice of pumpkin, 1 gm of *Yavakshara* and 12 gm of brown sugar to drink.

The following two prescriptions are particularly useful in dealing with enlargement of the prostate gland:

1. *Chandraprabha; Shweta Parpati; Yavakshara.*

   500 mg of *Chandraprabha*, 1 gm of *Shweta Parpati*, and 500 gm of *Yavakshara* to be taken thrice daily with decoction of *Gokharu.*

2. *Varunadi Lauha; Gokshuradyavaleha.*

   240 mg of *Varunadi Lauha* and 120 mg of *Gokshuradyavaleha* to be taken every twelve hours with cow's milk.

Home Remedies: Droppings of goat, and mud mixed with goat urine and saltpetre in equal quantities, should be mixed and used as a poultice on the bladder to induce greater flow of urine. A piece of thick woollen cloth, such as a blanket, may be dipped in cow's urine and the bladder should be fomented with it. Twenty grams of powder of cucumber seeds and 1 gm of salt may be mixed and taken with 200 ml of *Kanji*—a wine made of black carrots—to induce the flow of urine.

Diet and Other Regimen: Spices in the diet should be avoided. More liquids, preferably in the form of water, should be taken.

Fomentation of the pelvic region, particularly in the form of a Seitz bath, is recommended.

Syphilis *(Firanga)*

One of the most horrible venereal diseases, syphilis, is a contagious disease with a slow development.

Causes and Symptoms: Syphilis begins as a sore at the site of the infection, and in its tertiary stage, shows changes resembling those caused by leprosy and tuberculosis. In most cases, it is acquired through sexual intercourse with a person suffering from it. The two main types of syphilis are: acquired and inherited.

Acquired syphilis is caused by sexual intercourse with a person suffering from it, and sometimes, by contact with the sores or even the use of articles used by the patient such as utensils and clothes. The acquired form of the disease is commonly divided into three stages: primary, secondary, and tertiary. Sometimes these stages merge into one another and the disease proceeds as one long sequence of the various symptoms which appear as its severity increases. Sometimes the infection is so severe that ulcers appear all over the body. In other cases, it may appear only as a slight skin eruption but the effect on the constitution of the patient is no less harmful. The primary ulcers of syphilis are more like inflamed sores. At that stage, it is not very difficult to cure them if a proper diagnosis has been made. But the swelling subsides after some time and the inflamed lymphatic glands also show improvement. After a couple of months, however, the secondary symptoms start appearing in the form of a low fever, loss of appetite, vague pains throughout the body, and a faint red rash seen best upon the front of the chest. There may also be falling of hair, bloodlessness and sores in the mouth and the throat, headache, mental deterioration, and painful swelling on the bones of the body. There is also a general enlargement of the lymphatic glands.

The third or the tertiary stage develops after the lapse of a few months or even years, if the disease has remained untreated or inadequately treated. There is a growth of masses of granulated tissue all over the body. The patches of this growth known as 'gummata' may appear as hard nodules on the skin, or form tumour-like masses in the muscles, or cause great thickening of the bones, or they may develop in the brain or the spinal cord where their presence may show serious symptoms.

Still later effects are apt to follow, such as a disease of the arteries, leading to aneurysm, in which the artery dilates due to the yielding of the vessel wall and gradual stretching by the pressure of the blood; apoplexy or sudden paralysis; early mental failure; Locomotor ataxia, the disordered movement of the limbs in walking; and paralysis.

Inherited syphilis or congenital syphilis may affect the child before its birth. As a rule, this may lead to a miscarriage or a dead birth. If the child is born alive, he may start showing secondary symptoms after a few weeks. He may be deformed or become deaf. If the symptoms are suppressed for a few years, the child may develop a sunken nose, broad at the bridge, and may suffer from inflammation of the cornea or the iris.

The eruptions of syphilis may appear as painful boils on the prepuce of males or labia majora of the vagina among females. The eruptions turn into hard nodules called chancre and then subside, giving rise to other symptoms described above.

Medicines & Prescriptions: The following are the drugs of choice in the treatment of syphilis. Anyone or a combination of them may be taken.

1. *Savirvari.*	200 mg should be taken morning and evening with sweetened milk.
2. *Sarivadyavaleha.*	12 gm should be taken at breakfast time with milk.
3. *Sarivadyasava.*	20 mg should be taken with water after meals twice a day.
4. *Rasachandradi Yoga.*	A 500 mg capsule should be taken thrice daily.
5. *Hingulamrita Yoga.*	One teaspoonful to be taken thrice daily.

Diet and Other Regimen: A patient suffering from syphilis should be advised to take a salt-free diet as it helps in fast recovery. Bitter, sour, and pungent substances should be avoided.

Intercourse is strictly forbidden.

Chancre *(Dhwajabhanga)*

Chancre refers to the primary lesion of syphilis according to Allopathy, but in Ayurveda, it is treated separately.

Causes and Symptoms: Chancre is a contagious disease contacted through sexual intercourse with an infected person. According to Ayurveda, chancre is of five types: three varieties are borne out of the vitiation of the three different *doshas* of the body, one by the vitiation of the blood, and the fifth because of the vitiation of all the three different *doshas* together. Chancre is known as *Updansha* in Ayurveda but Charaka has described it as *Dhwajabhanga.*

Chancre is characterised by pain as if the affected part, generally the male organ or the outer vagina, is being pierced by a needle. Eruptions like small boils appear which exude pus of a pale yellow colour. In chancre born out of the vitiation of blood, there may be exudation of blood from the affected part. The variety of chancre caused by the vitiation of all the three *doshas* of the body is generally incurable.

When the boils burst, they give rise to wounds with sharply defined edges. The affliction spreads to the glans penis and the prepuce in the males, and the labia minora and clitoris in the females. There is also a feeling of itching and inflammation and the parts are tender to touch.

Medicines & Prescriptions: The following medicines are indicated in cases of chancre:

1. *Rasamanikya; Varadadi Guggul; Chopchina Churna.*	120 mg *Rasamanikya,* 1½ gm *Varadadi Guggul,* and 1½ gm *Chopchina Churna*—all to be taken twice daily with decoction of *neem* leaves.

2. *Chopchinadi Paka.*	12 mg to be taken once at breakfast time with milk.
3. *Sarivadyasava.*	12 ml to be taken with water after meals, twice daily.
4. *Rasashekhar.*	240 mg to be taken at bedtime with water.

Bhairava Ratnavali is a well-known preparation for chancre. It should be given in doses of 900 mg daily for 3 days and 300 mg for the next 11 days. The total intake should be about 5.1 gm in 14 days. The maximum allowed is 7.5 gm of the medicine throughout the course of the treatment. The medicine must be given in a capsule because its direct oral administration may lead to eruptions in the mouth.

Diet and Other Regimen: The dietary regimen is the same as has been recommended for patients suffering from syphilis.

Cleanliness of the pelvic region, particularly, of the male organ, should be strictly maintained. The affected parts should be washed with decoction of *neem* leaves and properly dried. Washing the affected areas with milk, and using hot water for cleaning the parts is also helpful.

Gonorrhoea *(Ushnavata)*

Gonorrhoea is an inflammatory disease affecting, especially, the mucous membrane of the urethra in the male, and that of the vagina in the female, but spreading to other parts of the body too.

Causes and Symptoms: Gonorrhoea is directly contagious, usually by sexual intercourse. However, it can occasionally be conveyed by discharge on towels or clothing as well.

In men, the disease manifests itself in the form of irritation of the urethra, scalding pain on passing urine, and a viscid, yellowish-white discharge. The lymph glands in the groin often become enlarged and may suppurate. The urine contains yellow threads of pus visible to the naked eye. When the disease continues for some time, inflammation in the neighbouring organs may appear—the testicles, prostate gland, and the bladder being affected. At a still later stage, the inflammation of the urethra is apt to lead to formation of fibrous tissue around it, leading to its narrowing, and great difficulty in passing urine. The infection may spread to the various joints of the body, making them stiff. Occasionally, general septicaemia with inflammation of the heart valves and abscesses in various parts of the body may also set in. Gonorrhoea may also cause a severe form of conjunctivitis, and in newly-born children, it may lead to total blindness. This condition is called ophthalmia neonatorum.

In females, the course and complications of the disease are somewhat different. It begins with a yellow vaginal discharge, pain on passing urine, and very often, inflammation of the glands situated close to the valva—the mouth of the vagina. The most serious problem is that the inflammation may spread to the uterus, the fallopian tubes, and the ovaries, causing permanent damage. Occasionally, it may lead to peritonitis, that is, inflammation of the enveloping membrane of the abdomen, with fatal results. Many cases of continued ill health, sterility, and recurring miscarriages are due to these changes.

Medicines & Prescriptions: The following medicines are recommended:

1. *Puyamehantaka Rasa; Raladi Churna.*	1 gm of *Puyamehantaka Rasa* and 3 gm of *Raladi Churna* to be taken thrice daily with water, or with water to which a little unboiled fresh milk is added.
2. *Chandanadi Vati.*	½ gm to be taken in two hourly doses along with the medicine prescribed above.
3. *Shatapatryadi Churna.*	4 gm to be taken in a single dose at night with warm cow's milk.

Along with the oral medication, local applications are advised. The urethra should be flushed with a solution of potassium permanganate—1:3,000—with the help of a syringe. The syringe may be kept in the urethra for five minutes before its contents are allowed to come out.

The medicines prescribed for dysuria are also effective in gonorrhoea.

Diet and Other Regimen: Spicy foods should be avoided. More liquids should be taken.

The patient should be given complete rest. Riding horses or other forms of transport, particularly in which the hips come in contact with a hard seat, is prohibited, as is any discussion or thinking of sex. Warm water baths are indicated. Diuretics and laxatives in case of constipation are also advised. Fluid intake should be increased—water mixed with a little milk being the chief drink.

Gynaecological Disorders *(Stree Rog)*

We shall now come to the diseases which are peculiar to females. Of them, the chief disorders are connected with menstruation, discharge or white liquid laced with pus, diseases connected with pregnancy and child birth, prolapse of the uterus, infertility, and frigidity. Let us first take the disorders connected with menstruation.

Menstruation is a periodic change occurring in females, and also in some higher apes, which consists of discharge of blood from the cavity of the womb. It begins between the ages of twelve to thirteen years in warm climates and later in cold regions. The duration of each menstrual period varies slightly from 28 to 30 days. The menstrual flow stops when a woman becomes pregnant, and stops completely around the age of forty-four or fifty years when it is known as the menopause or the grand climacteric.

The two main disorders relating to menstruation are: amenorrhoea (*nashtartava*) and dysmenorrhoea (*kashtartava*); and menorrhagia or metrorrhagia.

Amenorrhoea and Dysmenorrhoea
(Nashtartava and Kashtartava)

Amenorrhoea refers to an abnormal absence of menstruation or scanty discharge. Dysmenorrhoea is the term given to a painful or difficult menstruation.

Causes and Symptoms: Amenorrhoea or scanty discharge of menstrual blood may be due to anaemia or general ill health, or due to certain serious diseases like TB, Bright's disease, or malaria of a prolonged nature.

Dysmenorrhoea is characterised by colicky pain and there is also prostration and vomiting. If the pain precedes the menstrual period, it is due to irritation in the ovary and is generally accompanied by pain in the groin.

Another cause of dysmenorrhoea is inflammation of the various internal organs like the uterus, the ovaries, or the fallopian tubes, that is, those that connect the ovaries with the uterus. Sometimes, the disorder is due to nervous causes, in which case there are spasmodic pains.

In cases of scanty discharge of menstrual blood, the main cause should be diagnosed and removed. If it is due to anaemia, the treatment for anaemia is a prerequisite to the treatment of amenorrhoea. Aggravated dyspepsia, prolonged malaria, or Bright's disease should be treated first, in case they have given rise to scanty and painful discharge. In cases where the exact cause is not known, general tonics and remedies for improving the health of the patient should be administered.

Medicines & Prescriptions: Ayurveda prescribes the following medicines in cases of amenorrhoea and dysmenorrhoea:

1. *Raja Pravartini; Voladi Vati or Nashtapushpantaka Rasa.*

   500 mg *of Raja Pravartini,* and 500 mg of *Voladi Vati* or *Nashtapushpantaka Rasa* to be taken with decoction of black sesame, leaves of *Lasora,* and *gur.*

2. *Kumaryasava; Shuddha Tankana.*

   20 ml of *Kumaryasava* and 240 mg of *Shuddha Tankana* to be taken twice daily, preferably after meals.

Home Remedies: Another helpful remedy is a decoction of 18 gm of the root of the cotton tree, *Telia Geru*—6 gms, leaves of rose bush—6 gms, root of *Chaulai*—6 gms, and *gur*—24 gms with 750 ml of water. The decoction should be allowed to boil till one-eighth is left. It should be given once daily for three days.

Diet and Other Regimen: A nourishing diet with plenty of milk, fruit, and vegetables should be taken.

A medical check-up for evidence of any chronic infection or disease is necessary.

Menorrhagia and Metrorrhagia *(Rakta Pradara)*

Excessive discharge of blood during the monthly periods is known as **menorrhagia,** but when there is bleeding at irregular intervals, it is termed as **metrorrhagia.**

Causes and Symptoms: In Ayurveda, menorrhagia and metrorrhagia are called *Rakta Pradara*. These conditions may arise due to the imbalance of the hormones which is caused by the aggravation of *pitta* in the body. Abnormal growths in the uterus or other organs may also produce profuse bleeding. If bleeding continues for a long time, there may be giddiness, headache, pain in the calves, and restlessness—the common concomitants of anaemia. Menstruation may start with pain in the abdomen, the back, or the hips; the flow may be excessive, leaving the patient extremely weak.

Home Remedies: Seven tender leaves of the pomegranate tree and seven grains of rice, ground into a paste, and given to a patient for a month twice daily, act both as a curative as well as a preventive medicine for this condition.

Medicines and Prescriptions: *Praval Pishti* in doses of 75 mg each is given four times a day.

Ashoka (*Saraca indica*) and *Lodhra* (*Symplocos racemosa*) are the two drugs of choice in the treatment of this condition. Preparations like *Ashokarishta* and *Lodrasava* are widely prescribed.

Other prescriptions for the treatment of menorrhagia and metrorrhagia are given below:

1. *Pradararipi Rasa;*   240 mg each of *Pradararipi*
   Bol Parpati;   *Rasa* and *Bol Parpati*, and
   Chandanadi Churna.   1 gm of *Chandanadi*
                          Churna to be taken twice
                          daily with honey.

2. *Pradarantaka Lauha;* 240 mg of *Pradarantaka*
   Chandraprabha;   *Lauha*, 500 mg of
   Pushyanuga Churna.   *Chandraprabha*, and 1 gm
                          of *Pushyanuga Churna* to
                          be taken morning and
                          evening with decoction of
                          Kusha grass.

Diet and Other Regimen: Hot and spicy foods should be avoided; sugarcane juice, grapes, bananas, and pomegranates are particularly useful in this condition.

The patient should be given complete bedrest. Any form of strain is to be avoided. Worry and anger also tend to aggravate the condition and the patient should be kept in pleasant surroundings. The foot of the bed should be slightly raised and no pillow should be used. Sexual intercourse should be prohibited.

Leucorrhoea *(Shweta Pradara)*

Leucorrhoea or whites is a condition in which there is a whitish discharge from the vagina. It may be thick and viscid, and foul smelling if it is caused by some infection.

Causes and Symptoms: In addition to infection, some hormonal and metabolic disorders are also responsible for the condition.

Ayurveda considers that leucorrhoea is caused by the vitiation of *kapha*; it occurs commonly among weak, emaciated, and anaemic women. It can also be due to inflammation of the womb following childbirth, displacement of the uterus, or gonorrhoea. Among young females, it may be due to thread worms, as the result of general debility combined with lack of cleanliness or infections.

In addition to the whitish discharge from the vaginal tract, there is weakness. as well as pain in the lumbar region and the calves. A burning sensation may be present along with constipation. There appears to be a direct relationship of this disease with a nervous temperament. In a chronic form, leucorrhoea causes irritability. The patient develops black patches under the eyes. Late nights precipitate the attack.

Home Remedies: A proper diagnosis of the disease must be made and the cause removed. In addition to the medicines prescribed below, a regular douching of the genital tract with a decoction of the bark of the banyan tree or the fig tree is very helpful. A tablespoonful each of the powders of the bark of the two trees should be boiled in a litre of water till it is reduced to about half. Douching with the lukewarm decoction keeps the vaginal tract healthy and clean.

A home remedy used for this condition is to soak about 10 gm of dry coriander or *dhania* in 100 ml of water overnight, and to drink the water in the early morning. It gives relief in seven to ten days in most cases.

Medicines & Prescriptions: The medicine of choice for this condition is, of course, *Pradarantaka Lauha*, a compound of some calxes, of which iron is the most important. *Kumari* (*Aloe vera*) is another wonderful remedy for the condition: it tones up the tissues of the uterus and prevents the exudation of any abnormal fluids. *Lodhra* (*Symplocos racemosa*) bark is another substance, the decoction of which can be used for douching the vaginal tract of a leucorrhoea patient. Alum or *tankan* is also one of the drugs used in leucorrhoea. A proper course of treatment should be:

1. *Pradarantaka Lauha; Chandraprabha; Pushyanuga Churna.*   240 mg of *Pradarantaka Lauha*, 500 mg of *Chandraprabha*, and 1 gm of *Pushyanuga Churna* should be taken morning and evening with decoction of the root of *Kusha* grass.

| 2. *Yamani Shadava.* | 4 gm to be taken twice daily. |
| 3. *Ashokarishta.* | 20 ml to be taken twice daily along with medicine No. 2 above. |

Alternatively, the following prescription should be advised:

1. *Kukkutanda Twakbhasma; Yashada Bhasma; Powder of Amla.*	240 mg of *Kukkutanda Twakbhasma*, 120 mg of *Yashada Bhasma*, and 500 mg of powder of *Amla* to be taken in the morning and evening with honey.
2. *Chandraprabha; Triphala Powder.*	500 mg of *Chandraprabha*, and 3 gm of *Triphala* powder to be taken at midday and night with warm water.
3. *Darukadi Churna.*	6 gm may be taken last thing at night with cow's milk.

For patients suffering from neurasthenia along with leucorrhoea, *Ratnaprabha Vatika* should be given in 120 mg doses in the morning and evening.

Diet and Other Regimen: A strict dietary regimen is necessary. Fried and spicy foods are to be avoided, as are pickles and other savouries. The patient should be encouraged to chew betel nut (*supari*) after meals: it has a curative effect and also prevents the development of the disease.

The patient should avoid mental strain of all kinds. Late nights and sexual intercourse are to be avoided. A brisk early morning walk is helpful.

Childbirth Fever (Prasuti Jwara)

Childbirth fever, also called puerperal fever, was at one time one of the common causes for mortality among mothers. Of all the disorders that a woman is subject to after she has given birth to a child, this fever is the most common.

Causes and Symptoms: Childbirth fever is of various types and has grades of severity. After the birth of the child, the mother is specially liable, for several reasons, to contract any infectious disease to which she may be exposed. In the first place she is much weakened by the strain through which she has passed, and often, by the loss of a great quantity of blood. In the second place, the injuries incidental to childbirth produce raw surfaces in the genital tract from which absorption occurs very easily.

The symptoms of puerperal fever appear on the second or third day after labour. There is general discomfort and feverishness, rise of temperature, quickening of the pulse, and pain in the lumbar region. Inflammation of the pelvic region may also be present in some cases. The fever may rise further and if the infection is not controlled, peritonitis may set in, leading, in some cases, to a most serious condition known as septicaemia or general blood poisoning. In some cases, the symptoms may not be checked and death may occur because of the involvement of the heart.

In case the temperature goes beyond 39.4°C, cold compresses should be applied to reduce it. If the patient is very weak and complains of dizziness, a blood transfusion should be given.

Medicines & Prescriptions:

1. *Prataplankeshwar Rasa; Sanjivani; Shuddha Tankan.*	240 mg of *Prataplankeshwar*, and 120 mg each of *Sanjivani* and *Shuddha Tankan* should be taken thrice daily with juice of ginger and honey.
2. *Devadarbadi Quath.*	58 mg to be taken in one dose in the morning.
3. *Saubhagya Vati.*	240 ml to be taken twice during the day.
4. *Dashmularishta.*	20 ml to be taken after medicine No. 3 above, with water.

If the fever is very high, *Shri Jaimangal Rasa* should be given in place of *Sanjivani* at No. 1 above. If the fever continues for some days in spite of medication, *Putpakwavisham-jwarantaka Lauha* and *Vasantmalati* may be given in doses of 20 ml each, thrice daily.

Diet and Other Regimen: A woman suffering from childbirth fever must be given nutritious foods that can be digested easily. Milk with sugar should be the mainstay of her diet. Sour and astringent substances should be avoided.

Clean, healthy surroundings are a must for a woman suffering from childbirth fever. Complete rest is indicated. Her genitals must be properly douched with a weak solution of potassium permanganate to keep them clean.

Displacement of the Uterus *(Yoni Vyapagata)*

Of the other disorders of the female genitalia, the displacement of the uterus or the womb is probably the most disturbing.

Causes and Symptoms: The uterus is slung in the pelvic cavity and has freedom of movement backwards and forwards, and upwards and downwards. In most cases, its displacement is downwards; in this case, it is known as prolapse. In this condition, the uterus slips downwards in between the bowel and the bladder. In very serious cases, it may actually protrude out of the vagina. This condition occurs generally in older women—usually those who are stout, have a considerable amount of work to do, and have in childbirth suffered laceration of the parts that should support the uterus.

Prolapse of the uterus is one of the twenty *Yoni Vyapagatas* described by Charaka, Sushruta, and Vagabhatta. One of the teachers, Madhava, has categorised these disorders as: five belonging to the class of diseases produced by vitiation of *vayu*, five caused by vitiation of *pitta*, another five caused by vitiation of *kapha*, and the rest caused by the vitiation of all the three *doshas*. Prolapse of the uterus is a condition which is caused, among other things, by the vitiation of all the three *doshas* of the body and is not easy to deal with.

Medicines & Prescriptions:

1. *Vachadi Churna; Prasanna.*	3 gm of *Vachadi Churna* and 24 ml of *Prasanna* may be mixed and fried in about 5 gm of *ghee* and taken once daily.
2. *Raja Pravartani Vati* or *Bolaadi Vata* or *Rajodoshahari Vati.*	240 mg to be taken thrice daily.

When the condition has improved a little, tonics like *bhasmas* of gold, silver, or copper should be administered.

In some difficult cases, surgical intervention may be needed to repair the weakened parts that hold the uterus in its proper place.

Diet and Other Regimen: A light but nutritious diet is recommended.

The patient must be allowed to have rest; her movements should be restricted, and lifting of weights or vigorous work prohibited, as it is likely to aggravate the condition.

Sterility *(Vandhyatva)*

Sterility may be defined as the inability to conceive among females, and the failure or incapacity of a male to impregnate a female. The failure to reproduce, to give a broad definition of sterility, must be distinguished from frigidity among females and impotence among males. Frigidity and impotence both indicate a failure to perform the sex act or to perform it imperfectly. A female conceives when the sperm of the male, inserted into the vagina during the sexual intercourse, travels through the uterus and unites with the ovum secreted by the ovaries. If this union fails to occur, the woman does not conceive. If the seminal fluid of the male does not contain the sperms needed to impregnate the ova, he is said to be sterile.

Causes and Symptoms: According to ancient Ayurvedic texts, the general causes of sterility are: defective sperms or ova, congestion of the ovaries or the ducts which carry the sperm, trauma sustained by the genital organs, functional disorders of the reproductive organs, congenital defects in those organs, deformities resulting from injuries or certain diseases like syphilis or gonorrhoea, and improper development of the reproductive organs. We shall deal with sterility in females and males separately.

Sterility among Females: Sterility among females may be caused by certain congenital deformities such as the mouth of the uterus being clogged congenitally or by an inflammation, displacement of the uterus, inflammation of the mouth of the womb, anaemia and other diseases, malnutrition, and blood poisoning.

Congenital or organic defects in the reproductive organs can be cured only through surgery, but if sterility is due to functional causes, it is easy to cure. The vitiation of the various *doshas*—*vata*, *pitta*, and *kapha*—any one of them, or all the three together—is likely to lead to sterility.

Medicines & Prescriptions: The most effective remedy for sterility among females is *Phala Ghrita*. It should be given in doses of two teaspoonfuls each, twice daily, preferably on an empty stomach, with milk. Another drug of choice is *Vanga Bhasma*. It should be given in doses of 150 mg each, twice daily with honey. *Shilajit* is another effective drug in the treatment of this condition: it should be given in doses of one teaspoonful twice daily.

Bala (*Sida rhombifolia*) is used both internally and locally for the treatment of sterility. The root of this plant is boiled in milk and oil. It is used with lukewarm water as a douche. It removes the defects in the mucous membrane of the genital tract, which inhibit the effective union of the sperm with the ovum in the uterus. The medicated oil is given with a cup of milk in the morning in a dose of one teaspoonful.

The above medicines are to be administered after the physician is sure that the failure to conceive on the part of the woman is due to some defect in her genital organs. The best course is to ensure that the husband is not sterile: this can be done through an examination of his semen. Generally it is found that 35 per cent of the cases of sterility are due to weak or defective sperms. If that is the case, the male partner should be treated first.

Excessive fat often inhibits conception. Obesity must, in that case, be treated first through regulation of diet and a regimen of slimming exercises.

Diet and Other Regimen: A woman under treatment for sterility must be advised to desist from alkaline and pungent foods. Fruits and sweet substances should be consumed in larger quantities. The diet should be adequate to meet all the needs of the body. It must contain sufficient proteins.

Daily physical exercise and proper hygiene are recommended.

Sterility among Males: Sterility among males is the result of absence of sperm in the semen—a condition called azoospermia; or paucity of the sperms—oligospermia.

Sterility among males may be caused, as in the case of the females, by prolonged illness, a venereal disease, injuries, or congenital deformities. For example, if there is a malfunctioning of the ductless glands which secrete the hormones responsible for the regulation of the sperm, infertility or failure to procreate would definitely result.

It is necessary here to stress that sterility among males should not be confused with impotence. The former is the incapacity to reproduce, whereas the latter is the failure to perform the sexual act. An impotent man may become the father of many children because even his incapacity to complete the coitus may not deter the emission of sperms which may unite with the ovum to form the foetus.

If there is a complete lack of sperms in the semen--the condition termed as azoospermia--it is not an easy malady to cure. But if the sperms are present but are too few in number to be effective (oligospermia), there is not much difficulty in handling the condition.

Medicines & Prescriptions: *Ashwagandha* (*Withania somnifera*) is the drug of choice for male infertility. The fresh root of this wild plant smells like the urine of a horse, hence the name *Ashwagandha* (literally, the smell of the horse). When dried, the smell disappears and the drug can be taken without any difficulty. The powder of the dried root of the plant is taken in doses of one teaspoonful each, twice daily, with milk. Alternatively, it may be boiled with milk, and sugar may be added to it. It is, in that case, turned into a linctus and a teaspoonful of it can be taken twice daily, followed by milk. Another preparation, *Ashwagandharishta*—the basic ingredients being *Ashwagandha* and alcohol—may be given in doses of 100 ml each after meals.

Another useful remedy is *Kapi Kacchu* (*Mucuna pruriens*) which is prescribed for male sterility. The seeds outside the pods of this wild-growing creeper are powdered after being roasted, and a teaspoonful of the powder is administered twice daily with a cup of milk.

But the most celebrated of the remedies for sterility in Ayurveda is *Makaradhwaja*. Given in a 150 mg dose to the patient on an empty stomach, with half a teaspoonful of butter and half a teaspoonful of sugar, it has a miraculous effect.

In addition, all the drugs prescribed for impotence are helpful in dealing with male sterility. But aphrodisiacs--drugs which stimulate sex—should be taken in proper quantities.

Diet and Other Regimen: The patient should be advised to desist from sour and pungent substances as they have a detrimental effect on the production of sperms. Milk, *ghee*, butter, and sweet substances are good for this condition. A high protein diet, particularly fish, white meat, and eggs, is recommended.

A man under treatment for sterility should avoid over-indulgence in sex.

Impotence *(Klaibya)*

Impotence is a disease peculiar to males; in females the corresponding disorder is known as frigidity. Impotence can be defined as the inability to perform the sexual act, or incomplete performance which leaves the female partner partially or totally dissatisfied.

Causes and Symptoms: Impotence may be partial or total, temporary or permanent. But the most satisfactory classification of the disorder is in either of two categories: organic or functional. Among organic causes are lesions of the external genitals, such as a tight foreskin; disturbances of the endocrine glands, such as diabetes, diminished activity of the gonads, thyroid gland, or the pituitary gland; diseases of the central nervous system, such as tabes dorsalis—a paralysing condition caused by syphilis; locomotor ataxia, or the disordered and disjointed movement of the limbs, due to lack of coordination; any severe disturbance of health, such as diabetes mellitus, addiction to alcohol and the like. Among the psychological factors are ignorance, fear, and weakness of sexual desire.

Ayurveda maintains that impotence may be caused by the vitiation of any of the three *doshas* of the body— *vata*, *pitta*, and *kapha*, or a combination of all the three.

It has been found that about seventy per cent of males complaining of the incapacity to perform the sexual act suffer from psychological impotence. They may be suffering from a guilt complex because of having indulged in masturbation in their childhood and adolescence, or they may be feeling guilty because they have been indulging in unnatural sex. Some of them may be in a perennially excited state due to constant thinking about performing the sexual act, and the moment they get an opportunity, they ejaculate even before their female partners have reached a state of physical readiness, or before the commencement of the act. Actual physical or organic impotence is rather rare.

Sushruta and Charaka have categorised impotent males according to the perversion that excites them to perform sexual activity. Sushruta has described them as *Aasekya*—those who are excited on licking the semen; *Saugandhika*—those who get excited when they smell the vagina; *Kumbhika*—those who get excited only when they are the passive partners in anal sex; and *Irshyaka*—those who are voyeurs and get excited when they watch others performing the sexual act. Charaka has

211

similarly classified impotent males according to their peculiar preferences.

Medicines & Prescriptions: In the case of organic impotence, such as a tight foreskin, surgery is the only recourse. If the failure to perform is psychological, a proper explanation of the facts of life to the patient would help.

In Ayurveda, *vajikarana* or aphrodisiacs have been developed from the earliest times to deal with cases of impotence. Drugs prescribed for sterility would definitely help.

The popular medicines used in the treatment of this condition according to *Bhiskharma Siddhi*, a popular treatise on Ayurvedic medicine, are: *Apatyakara Swarasa, Kamalakshadi Churna, Vanari Gutika, Shri Madananda Modaka, Mahachandanadi Taila, Mritsanjivani Sura, Virya Stambha Vati, Chandrodaya Rasa* and *Makaradhwaja*.

The medicines must, of course, be taken under the guidance of a qualified Ayurvedic physician as their indiscriminate use may lead to over-indulgence which may, in the final analysis, prove to be more harmful than the condition for which they have been taking a cure.

Diet and Other Regimen: A high protein diet is an essential part of the treatment. Fish, eggs, testicles of a goat, partridge meat, eggs of a crocodile, *urad dal*, butter, and *ghee* are specially recommended for impotency.

Mental tension should be avoided. If one is suffering from diabetes or taking any drugs for hypertension, the doctor should be consulted.

Frigidity *(Kaam Shauthalya)*

Frigidity, which literally means coldness, is a female disorder. A normal woman has a normal desire for sex. When the desire is absent or is feeble, or there is an antipathy towards the sexual act, the woman is said to be frigid.

Causes and Symptoms: Frigidity may be due to organic or functional reasons. Among the organic reasons are the diseases of the genital organs which inhibit the desire for sex.

Prolapse of the uterus or other abnormalities of the female genitalia can lead to a diminution of the desire for the sexual act. Frigidity may be caused by a trauma, such as rape or submission unwillingly to a person under some form of coercion. Inexpert handling by the male partner may also lead to frigidity. Sometimes, frigidity may be due to cultural reasons; the woman may feel that it is sinful to think of sexual union. This is, not infrequently, the case in our country where religious beliefs persuade women to suppress their natural urge for sex.

Medicines & Prescriptions: In case frigidity is due to a psychological cause, a psychological approach is the best way to deal with it. The patient must be taken into confidence and the facts of life explained to her. If the malady can be traced to any physical causes, they must be removed first before any improvement can be expected. If it is due to psychological reasons, a psychological approach is the best.

In other cases, aphrodisiacs may be helpful. The cause of the condition must be established before any treatment is started. Mental tension should be avoided.

Rasayana: The Key to Rejuvenation

स्वर्गतारारताम्राणि नागवंगौ च तीक्ष्णकम् ।
धातवः सप्त विज्ञेया अष्टमश्चपि पारदः ॥

Gold, silver, brass, lead, tin, iron, and copper are the seven metals used in medicine and mercury is supposed by some to be the eighth.

BHOJARATNAKAR

GERIATRICS IS that branch of medicine which deals with disorders and diseases associated with old age. In spite of the fact that modern medicine claims to have made a lot of progress in fighting disease, this branch of medicine is comparatively new. The increase in longevity due to the progress of medicine is posing a new problem, namely, that of dealing with people who are old and who, in spite of the fact that they are healthy, face certain problems that come with advancing age. Senile degeneration of certain organs of the body and blunting of the senses make life difficult, if not miserable, even though there may not be any morbidity, clinically speaking.

The Role of *Rasayana*

In Ayurveda, *rasayana* is a well-developed science. Literally, *rasayana* means the augmentation of *rasa*, the vital fluid produced by the digestion of food, which sustains the body through the strengthening of the *dhatus*. It is the *rasa* flowing in the body which sustains life: when it stops flowing, life comes to an end. *Rasayana* is, therefore, the medium

214

through which the *rasa* is maintained, freshened, and augmented. According to Sushruta, *Rasayana Shastra* is a part of Ayurveda and its aims are: to increase longevity to 100 years, to increase it to more than 100 years, to increase the power of the brain, to improve health and to make a person more active, to remove all morbidity from the body, and to maintain the youth of the individual.

Another Acharya, Vagabhatta, says: *Rasayana* is the medium through which age can be increased as well as the vigour, as also the brain power, youth, and zeal of the individual. Charaka has also commented on *Rasayana Shastra* in a similar vein.

Another connotation of *rasa,* which follows from the first, is that it is a medicine which will maintain the life and health of the individual, and increase his bodily and mental vigour. Medicines are categorised according to whether they promote general health and longevity, sexual vigour, or fight disease. The first category is that of *rasayana*, the second of *vajikarana*, and the third of *aushadhis* or medicines. These categories are not mutually exclusive, because some of the *aushadhis* may act as *rasayanas* and vice versa.

Rasayana ensures complete health to the individual, ensures a long life for him, and sharpens his intelligence to such an extent that a single reading would suffice for him to commit something to memory. It gives a celestial glow to the body, and endows it with godly vigour and lightning-like alacrity. For example, if *Rasayana Chyavanaprasha* is taken over a long period regularly, it rids the body of all types of morbidity, promotes mental and somatic vigour, and ensures a long life. The sages of old who lived long, disease-free, and vigorous lives,did so with the help of *rasayanas.* Lord Indra is supposed to have given the knowledge of these panaceas to the sages. The *rasayanas* of which Lord Indra spoke were based on such drugs as *Endri, Brahmi, Kakoti, Kshirpushpi, Shravani, Mahashravani, Shatavari, Vadarikanda, Jeevanti, Punarnava, Sthira, Vacha, Chhatra, Atichattra, Meda* and countless others.

Rasayanas prepared from *Amalaki, Haritiki, Triphala, Bhringaraja, Ashwagandha, Punarnava, Chitraka* and many other drugs have been used from time immemorial and have been instrumental in giving long, disease-free, and vigorous lives to their users.

Bhasmas as Medicines

In addition to *rasayanas*, Ayurveda has taken recourse to use of metals, jewels, and pearls as medicines. These elements are turned into calxes or *bhasmas* for administration in different diseases. The human body contains some chemical elements which are known as trace elements, that is, elements whose mere traces are to be found in the human body. The trace elements are distributed throughout the tissues of the body in very small amounts and are essential for the nutrition of the body. Nine such elements are now recognised: cobalt, copper, fluorine, iodine, iron, manganese, molybdenum, selenium, and zinc. No wonder Ayurveda has always taken recourse to calxes of precious and other metals for dealing with certain deficiency diseases. Calxes of gold, silver, copper, and iron are widely used.

Jewels or *ratnas* include precious and semi-precious stones which are turned into calxes and used as drugs because of their therapeutic properties. Major jewels or *maharatnas* include: diamond—*hiraka*; ruby—*manikya*; pearl—*mukta*; topaz—*pushparaga*; sapphire—*neelam*; emerald—*tarksha*; cat's eye—*vaidurya*; zircon—*gomedak;* and coul—*vidruma. Uparatnas* or minor jewels are: turmulin—*vaikranta*; sun-stone—*suryakanta*; moonstone—*chandrakanta*; lapis lazuli—*rajavarta*; turquoise—*pheroza*; and crystal—*sphatika.*

Calxes of these stones are formed by following the correct pharmaceutical procedures like that of tituration and repeated heating. They are then ground into fine powders. Minute doses, even 50 mg of these preparations, are given for the amelioration of morbid conditions; for purposes of *vajikarana*, that is, increasing sexual vigour; and rejuvenation.

The various calxes have different properties: for example, in cases of severe anaemia or blood loss due to injuries, *Lauha Bhasma* (calx of iron) is given. It is just like a modern physician giving iron tablets to his patients, the only difference being that *Lauha Bhasma* is more readily assimilated into the system, whereas the fersolate tablets are passed through the stool because the system cannot absorb iron in that raw and rough shape. The calx of diamond is a powerful cardiac tonic and one of the best elixirs. It is helpful in curing diabetes, urinary troubles, anaemia, oedema, and even impotence, because it is a powerful aphrodisiac. The calx of rubies promotes intelligence, virility, longevity; and also cures disorders produced by the vitiation of the three *doshas*, including consumption. The calx of pearls has a cooling effect on the system and cures the burning sensation in various parts of the body, fevers, and chronic urinary infections. It also promotes growth of bones and the teeth, and is an anti-toxin. The calx of topaz has a cooling and carminative effect. It promotes digestion and is used in certain serious afflictions of the skin like leprosy and other disorders caused by the aggravation of *vata* and *kapha*. It is also useful in cases where the patients are unable to put on weight in spite of a normal diet. The calx of sapphire promotes virility and digestion; ensures a healthy complexion; and is a wonderful remedy in cases of a fistula, piles, skin diseases like leprosy, and pulmonary afflictions like asthma and bronchitis. The calx of emerald is a known remedy for providing immunity against disease and is helpful in cases of anaemia, oedema, and other disorders caused by the vitiation of all the three *doshas*. The calx of cat's eye is a laxative and promotes digestion and eye-sight. It also helps in stopping haemorrhages and disorders attendant upon aggravation of *pitta*. *Gomeda* is a carminative and helps in dealing with disorders of the digestion like anorexia. Coral is alkaline and promotes digestion and virility. It is also an anti-toxin and is a wonderful remedy for night sweats.

It is in the sphere of *rasayanas* and the various *bhasmas* that Ayurveda has proved its superiority. Maintenance of bodily and mental vigour—the main objective of *rasayana*—is possible only through recourse to Ayurveda.

The Origin of
Charaka Samhita & *Sushruta Samhita*

The *Charaka Samhita*, a detailed treatise on Ayurveda–the ancient system of medicine, elucidates the traditional story about the origin of Ayurveda.

Once, in an assembly of about fifty eminent sages, the topic of discussion revolved around getting rid of prevailing diseases which were causing irreparable harm to human beings. The conclave of sages made an unanimous decision to seek the advice of Lord Indra who had imbibed the secret of longevity.

In actuality, Brahma, the Creator, had imparted this knowledge to Prajapati Daksha, who, in turn, had passed it on to the two Ashwinikumaras. The latter had then communicated this science in its entirety to Lord Indra.

Thus it happened that Sage Bharadwaja was chosen to approach Lord Indra. Bowing humbly before him, he pleaded, 'Diseases have arisen which are a terror to all human beings. Tell me, O Lord of the Immortals, the appropriate means of curing them.'

Lord Indra was aware of the vast knowledge and wisdom that Sage Bharadwaja himself possessed and was hence able to instruct him in Ayurveda in no time at all.

On his return, Bharadwaja shared his newly-found knowledge with the other sages, one of whom was Punarvasu Atreya. Atreya tutored his own six disciples on the subject, which they condensed into treatises to mitigate the human suffering. One of the better treatises was authored by Agnivesha and entitled *Agnivesha Tantra*. This handbook was enlarged and revised by Charaka around the first century A.D. and hence came to be known as the *Charaka Samhita*.

Between the seventh and ninth centuries A.D., the *Charaka Samhita* was acknowledged as an authority on medicine in the Islamic and Roman worlds. During the ninth century A.D., the book was revised by a Kashmiri *pundit* named Dridhabala. The *Charaka Samhita*, in its present form, is thus the handiwork of Dridhabala.

Divided into eight sections, the treatise not only imparts knowledge about Ayurveda in its totality, but also explains the logic and philosophy on which this system of medicine is based.

The *Sushruta Samhita* deals with the surgical aspects of Ayurveda. Sushruta is believed to have lived around the sixth century B.C. and is said to have imbibed his knowledge from Dhanwantari. Sushruta's original work seems to have been revised and supplemented by Nagarjuna between the third and fourth centuries A.D.

The *Charaka Samhita* and the *Sushruta Samhita* are, therefore, the most widely accepted authoritative works on Ayurveda–the *Charaka Samhita* expounding the practice and philosophy of the ancient system of medicine, while the *Sushruta Samhita* is concerned with its surgical aspects.

The Medical Oath of *Charaka*

To practice Ayurvedic medicine in ancient India, seven years of intense, disciplined studies in eight different branches of Ayurveda were required. On successful completion of the course, the student was further required to reaffirm his dedication to the 'Science of Living' by taking the following solemn oath:*

Day and night however thou mayest be engaged, thou shalt endeavour for the relief of the patient with all thy heart and soul. Thou shalt not desert or injure the patient even for the sake of thy life or thy living. Thou shalt not commit adultery even in thought. Thou shalt not covet others' possessions. Thou shalt be modest in thy attire and appearance. Thou should not be a drunkard or a sinful man, nor shouldst thou associate with the abettors of crimes.

Thou shouldst speak words that are gentle, pure and righteous, pleasing, worthy, true, wholesome and moderate. Thy behaviour must be in consideration of time and place and heedful of past experience. Thou shalt act always with a view to the acquisition of knowledge.

No persons who are hated by the king, or who are haters of the king; or who are hated by the public, or who are haters of the public shall receive treatment. Similarly, those that are of very unnatural, wicked and miserable character and conduct; those who have not vindicated their honour; and those who are on the point of death; and similarly, women who are unattended by their husbands or guardians shall not receive treatment.

No offering of meat by a woman without the knowledge of her husband or guardian shall be accepted by thee. While entering the patient's house, thou shalt be accompanied by a man who is known

---

* As given in *Charaka Samhita*, a compendium on Ayurveda authored by Charaka—a renowned authority on Ayurvedic medicine who lived sometime between the 2nd century B.C. and 2nd century A.D.

to the patient and who has his permission to enter, and thou shalt be well-clad and bent of head, self-possessed, and conduct thyself after repeated consideration. Thou shalt thus properly make thy entry. Having entered, thy speech, mind, intellect and senses shall be entirely devoted to no other thought than that of being helpful to the patient and of things concerning him only. The peculiar customs of the patient's household shall not be made public. Even knowing that the patient's lifespan has come to its close, it shall not be mentioned by thee there, where, if so done, it would cause shock to the patient or to others.

Though possessed of knowledge, one shouldst not boast very much of his knowledge. Most people are offended by the boastfulness of even those who are otherwise good and well-informed.

There is no limit at all to which the knowledge of Ayurveda can be acquired, so thou shouldst apply thyself to it with diligence. This is how thou shouldst act. Again, thou shouldst learn the skill of practice from another without carping. The entire world is the teacher to the intelligent and the foe to the unintelligent. Hence, knowing this well, thou shouldst listen and act according to the words of instruction of even an unfriendly person, when they are worthy and such as bring fame to you and long life, and are capable of giving you strength and prosperity.

Glossary

Addison's Disease: A disease characterized by progressive anaemia and debility, and brown discoloration of the skin.

Agnis: These are digestive juices, thirteen in number, that facilitate assimilation of food into *dhatus.*

Anabolism: The energy storing part of metabolism, the energy using part being called ketabolism.

Anaphylactic: Hypersensitivity of tissues to a dose of antigen, as a reaction against a previous dose.

Anorexia: A lack of appetite for food.

Arteriosclerosis: The loss of elasticity and thickening of the walls of the arteries.

Asphyxia: A lack of oxygen in the blood, causing unconsciousness or death.

Carminative: A drug or substance that relieves flatulence.

Catabolism: The breakdown of complex molecules in living organisms to form simpler ones with the release of energy.

Coryza: A catarrhal inflammation of the mucous membrane in the nose; a cold in the head; any disease with this as a symptom.

Cretinisns: Deformity or mental retardation due to thyroid deficiency.

Decoction: A process of boiling down so as to extract some essence.

Deha-Prakriti: A pre-determined body constitution that a person is born with, in which there is a predominance of *vata*, *pitta*, or *kapha*, or a combination of them.

Dementia Praecox: (See schizophrenia).

Dhatus: Seven body constituents: *rasa* (food juices), *rakta* (haemoglobin content of the blood), *mamsa* (muscle tissue), *medas* (fat tissue), *asthi* (bone tissue), *majja* (bone marrow), and *shukra* (semen).

Dyspnoea: Difficult or laboured breathing.

Exopthalmic Goitre: Protrusion of the eyeball due to increased activity of thyroid gland.

Haemoglobinuria: The presence of blood pigment in the urine.

Hyperpyrexia: High fever.

Jwara: Fever.

Kapha: One of the *tridoshas,* it comprises 5 types: *kledaka, avalambaka, bodhaka kapha, tarpaka,* and *shleshaka kapha.*

Linctus: A syrupy medicine, such as a soothing cough mixture.

Locomotor Ataxia: The loss of full control off bodily movements.

Malas: By-products of the *dhatus,* partly used by the body, and partly excreted as waste matter.

Myxoedema: A syndrome caused by hypothyroidism, resulting in thickening of the skin, weight gain, mental dullness, loss of energy, and sensitivity to cold.

Neuritis: Inflammation of a nerve or nerves.

Oja: The vital essence in the body.

Orchitis: Inflammation of the testicles.

Palliative: Anything used to alleviate pain, anxiety.

Pancha Bhutas: The *five* basic elements which the universe is composed of, namely, *prithvi* (earth), *ap* (water), *teja* (fire), *vayu* (air), and *akash* (ether).

Pancha Karma: Five methods of purification of the body.

Pathyapathya: The do's and don'ts of diet in Ayurveda.

Pitta: One of the *tridoshas,* it comprises 5 kinds: *paachak, ranjaka, sadhaka, alochaka,* and *bhrajaka.*

Poultice: A soft, medicated and usually heated mass applied to the body and kept in place with muslin etc, for relieving soreness and inflammation.

Pthisis: Chronic tuberculosis of the lungs.

Pyelonephritus: Inflammation of the kidney where urine is produced.

Rasa: This refers to taste which may be sweet, sour, saline, pungent, bitter and astringent.

Rasayana: The system of rejuvenation.

Rhinitis: Inflammation of the mucous membrane of the nose.

Rigor: Shivering.

Septicemia: Blood poisoning.

Strotas: Channels through which blood flows.

Suprarenal (glands): Glands situated above the kidneys.

Syncope: A temporary loss of consciousness caused by a fall in blood pressure.

Schizophrenia: A mental disease marked by a breakdown in the relation between thought, feeling and actions; frequently accompanied by delusion and retreat from social life. It is also known as Dementia Praecox.

Tridoshas: An important derivative of digestion and assimilation of food, the *tridoshas* comprise *vata, pitta* and *kapha.*

Triple Antigen: Three antigens, namely, of whooping cough, diphtheria and tetanus, whose injection protects against these diseases.

Thrombosis: The coagulation of the blood in a blood vessel or organ, causing a clot.

Thyrotoxicoses: A disease which results from an increase in the secretion of the thyroid gland.

Tetany: A disease with intermittent muscular spasms caused by malfunction of the parathyroid glands and a consequent deficiency of calcium.

Uraemia: A morbid condition due to the presence of urinary matter in the blood, normally eliminated by the kidneys.

Vajikarana: The system of increasing sexual stamina.

Vata: One of the *tridoshas,* and comprising five types: *prana, udana, vyana, samana, and apana.*